Fibrin Sealing in Surgical and Nonsurgical Fields

Volume **3**

G. Schlag J. Holle (Eds.)

Plastic Surgery Nerve Repair Burns

With 51 Figures, Some in Color, and 23 Tables

Springer-Verlag
Berlin Heidelberg New York
London Paris Tokyo
Hong Kong Barcelona
Budapest

Univ.-Prof. Dr. GÜNTHER SCHLAG
Ludwig-Boltzmann-Institut
für experimentelle und klinische Traumatologie
Donaueschingenstraße 13, 1200 Wien, Austria

Univ.-Prof. Dr. JÜRGEN HOLLE
Wilhelminenspital
Abteilung für Plastische und
Wiederherstellungschirurgie
Montleartstraße 37, 1160 Wien, Austria

ISBN 3-540-58550-8 Springer-Verlag Berlin Heidelberg New York

Library of Congress Cataloging-in-Publication Data.
Plastic surgery, nerve repair, burns / G. Schlag (ed.). p. cm. – (Fibrin sealing in surgical and nonsurgical fields ; v. 3) Includes index. ISBN 3-540-58550-8 (alk. paper). 1. Fibrin tissue adhesive. 2. Surgery, Plastic. 3. Nerves, Peripheral – Wounds and injuries – Surgery. 4. Burns and scalds – Treatment. I. Schlag, Günther. II. Series. [DNLM: 1. Surgery, Plastic. 2. Neurosurgery – methods. 3. Burns – therapy 4. Fibrin Tissue Adhesive. WO 600 P7142 1995]
RD73.F52F53 1994 vol. 3 [RD73.F52] 617.1'406 s–dc20 [617'.9178]

Production: PRO EDIT GmbH, D-69126 Heidelberg
Typesetting: Mitterweger, D-68723 Plankstadt
SPIN: 10476790 23/3130 5 4 3 2 1 0 – Printed on acid-free paper

Preface

These eight volumes, which developed out of the international congress "Update and Future Trends in Fibrin Sealing in Surgical and Nonsurgical Fields" held in November 1992, present the state of the art in fibrin sealing. Initially, fibrin sealant played an important role in surgery. During the past few years, it has been increasingly applied nonsurgically and we can now say that it has become an integral component of medical treatment.

The doubts which have been raised by nonusers about the efficacy of fibrin sealant are no longer valid. The correct indication and technique continue to be basic prerequisites for effective treatment. Even today – 20 years after fibrin sealant was first used – the three most prominent effects of fibrin sealant are still hemostasis, sealing of the wound, and support of wound healing.

The problems posed by the transmission of viral infections have gained substantially in importance because of the potential transmission of AIDS via fibrin sealant. Fortunately, this is so unlikely today that it no longer represents a cause for concern, which does not mean, however, that research in this field can be discontinued.

Seven years have passed since the last series of books on fibrin sealing were published. Since then many new results have been obtained and clear indications for the use of fibrin glue have developed. Fibrin sealant has found new applications in plastic surgery for optimal local hemostasis of large wound surfaces, for sealing of autologous implants, and to seal large bleeding surfaces. Fibrin sealant is also being used successfully in the treatment of hemangioma, with or without magnesium implants. Another new indication is the use of fibrin sealant in cosmetic surgery of the nose to fix autologous cartilage and bone implants, but also for local hemostasis and optimal adaptation of the soft parts of the nose to the framework.

Fibrin sealant has been applied successfully for many years in face lifting to prevent swelling and bleeding. Another indication is in Dupuytren's contracture, where it has improved healing rates and reduced postoperative morbidity.

Fibrin sealant has been applied in experimental studies in nerve repair both as a conduit and as a matrix for gap healing in silicon conduits in peripheral nerve repair with promising results. The original chains of blockage by fibrin sealant between two nerve ends could be disproved, because gaps of 4 mm have been bridged in nerve regeneration. In clinical treatment fibrin sealant seems to have a strong role in peripheral nerve repair, although there is no difference in the efficacy compared to sutures. Fibrin sealing does, however, reduce the operation time and facilitates nerve sprouting across junction interfaces, with a slightly lower total time of regeneration.

In the management of deep burns with fibrin sealant particularly good hemostasis and improved wound healing have been observed. In head and neck burns better cosmetic results have been obtained.

Fibrin sealing has also been applied successfully in tangential excisions of burn wounds for hemostasis and securing of autografts, and blood loss has been markedly reduced, too. Culture of autologous keratinocytes with fibrin sealant to cover burn wounds is an interesting prospect for the future. Very promising results have been reported.

We, the editors, would like to thank all the authors for their cooperation and excellent contributions and photographs. Their work has made publication of these eight volumes on fibrin sealing possible. Special thanks are due to Dr. V. Gebhardt and his expert colleagues for efficient and constructive cooperation in the publication of these books at the Springer publishing company and to Gudrun Schrodt for her untiring efforts in obtaining manuscripts, proof reading, and corresponding with the authors.

G. SCHLAG
J. HOLLE

Contents

I. Plastic Surgery

II. Nerve Repair

III. Burns

List of Contributors

Adant, J. P.
Department of Maxillofacial and Plastic Surgery,
University of Liège, CHU, Sart Tilman, 4000 Liège, Belgium

Arioli, N.
Division of Plastic Surgery, Istituto Nazionale Tumori,
Via Venezian 1, 20133 Milan, Italy

Arturson, G.
Burn Centre and Department of Plastic and Hand Surgery,
University Hospital, 75185 Uppsala, Sweden

Basse-Catalinat, B.
CHU Pellegrin-Tondu, Place Amélie Raba-Léon,
33000 Bordeaux, France

Baudet, J.
CHU Pellegrin-Tondu, Place Amélie Raba-Léon,
33000 Bordeaux, France

Berdalle, J.-P.
Service des Brûlés, CHU de Tours, Hôpital Trousseau,
37044 Tours Cedex, France

Blache, C.
University of South Alabama, Burn Center, College of Medicine,
2451 Fillingim Street, Mobile, AL 36617-2293, USA

Boeckx, W.
Plastic and Reconstructive Surgery, University Ziekenhuizen,
Herestraat 49, 3000 Leuven, Belgium

Bonnard, C.
Clinique Longeraie and University Hospital,
9 Avenue de la Gare, 1003 Lausanne, Switzerland

Bori, R.
Centro Médico Teknon, M. de Vilallonga, 12,
08017 Barcelona, Spain

Bouccara, D.
Service d'Oto-Rhino-Laryngologie, Hôpital Beaujon,
Faculté de Médecine Xavier Bichat, Université Paris 7,
100, Bvd. Général Leclerc, 92110 Clichy, France

Calabrese, L.
Division of Head and Neck Surgery, Istituto Nazionale Tumori,
Via Venezian 1, 20133 Milan, Italy

D'Silva, M.
Department of General and Abdominal Surgery, CHU,
Sart Tilman, 4000 Liège, Belgium

Danielsson, P.
Department of Plastic Surgery, Hand Surgery and Burns,
University Hospital of Linköping, 85185 Linköping, Sweden

Detroz, B.
Department of General and Abdominal Surgery, CHU,
Sart Tilman, 4000 Liège, Belgium

Dhennin, Ch.
Service des Brûlés, CHU de Tours, Hôpital Trousseau,
37044 Tours Cedex, France

Dioguardi, D.
Institute of Plastic Surgery, University of Bari,
Policlinic, 70124 Bari, Italy

Dyess, D. L.
University of South Alabama, Burn Center, College of Medicine,
2451 Fillingim Street, Mobile, AL 36617-2293, USA

Eberlin, J. L.
27, route de Frontenais, 2900 Porrentruy, Switzerland

Fabrizio, T.
Division of Plastic Surgery, S. Anna General Hospital,
Via Napoleona 60, 22100 Como, Italy

Feauveaux, J.-F.
Service des Brûlés, CHU de Tours, Hôpital Trousseau,
37044 Tours Cedex, France

Fini, M.
Experimental Surgery, Istituto di Ricerca Codivilla Putti I.O.R.,
Via di Barbiano 1/10, 40136 Bologna, Italy

Fletcher, J. R.
University of South Alabama, Burn Center, College of Medicine,
2451 Fillingim Street, Mobile, AL 36617-2293, USA

GIARDINO, R.
Experimental Surgery, Istituto di Ricerca Codivilla Putti I.O.R.,
Via di Barbiano 1/10, 40136 Bologna, Italy

GIAVARESI, G.
Experimental Surgery, Istituto di Ricerca Codivilla Putti I.O.R.,
Via di Barbiano 1/10, 40136 Bologna, Italy

GITT, H. A.
Department of Dermatology/Dermatosurgery,
Universität Leipzig, Liebigstraße 21, 04177 Leipzig, Germany

GRABOSCH, A.
Plastic Surgery and Handsurgery, Mauerstraße 65,
10117 Berlin, Germany

GUELINCKX, P.
Plastic and Reconstructive Surgery, University Ziekenhuizen,
Herestraat 49, 3000 Leuven, Belgium

HEDLUND, A.
Burn Centre and Department of Plastic and Hand Surgery,
University Hospital, 751 85 Uppsala, Sweden

HIRGSTETTER, C.
Universitätsklinik und Poliklinik der TU München,
Handchirurgie, Klinikum Rechts der Isar,
Ismaninger Straße 22, 81664 München, Germany

HORCH, R.
Sektion Plastische Chirurgie, Universität Freiburg,
Hugstetter Str. 55, 79106 Freiburg, Germany

HU, W.
CHU Pellegrin-Tondu, Place Amélie Raba-Léon,
33000 Bordeaux, France

JULIEN, N.
Service d'Oto-Rhino-Laryngologie, Hôpital Beaujon,
Faculté de Médecine Xavier Bichat, Université Paris 7,
100, Bvd. Général Leclerc, 92110 Clichy, France

KAISER, H. W.
Department of Dermatology, Universität Bonn,
Sigmund-Freud-Straße 25, 53105 Bonn, Germany

KOPP, J.
Plastic and Hand Surgery Section, Universität Freiburg,
Hugstetter Straße 55, 79106 Freiburg, Germany

KRÜGER, A.
Plastic and Reconstructive Operations, Salvatorweg 12,
47051 Duisburg, Germany

LECLERCQ, P.
Centre des Grands Brûlés IMTR, 6280 Loverdal, Belgium

LEDOUX, M.
Centre des Grands Brûlés IMTR, 6280 Loverdal, Belgium

LEICHTFRIED, G.
Ludwig Boltzmann Institute for Experimental and Clinical Traumatology,
Donaueschingenstraße 13, 1200 Vienna, Austria

LORENZO, J. C.
Pathology Department, Hospital San Rafael,
Copérnico, 37, 08021 Barcelona, Spain

LUTERMAN, A.
University of South Alabama, Burn Center, College of Medicine,
2451 Fillingim Street, Mobile, AL 36617-2293, USA

MEYER, V. E.
Division of Hand, Plastic and Reconstructive Surgery,
Department of Surgery, University Hospital Medical School,
8091 Zürich, Switzerland

MOLINARI, R.
Division of Head and Neck Surgery, Istituto Nazionale Tumori,
Via Venezian 1, 20133 Milan, Italy

NARAKAS, A. O.†
Clinique Longeraie and University Hospital,
9, Avenue de la Gare, 1003 Lausanne, Switzerland

NATOWITZ, L.
Department of General and Abdominal Surgery, CHU,
Sart Tilman, 4000 Liège, Belgium

NAVA, M.
Division of Plastic Surgery, Istituto Nationale Tumori,
Via Venezian 1, 20133 Milan, Italy

NICOLI ALDINI, N.
Experimental Surgery, Istituto di Ricerca Codivilla Putti I.O.R.,
Via di Barbiano 1/10, 40136 Bologna, Italy

NOËL, X.
Clinique Tourny, Rue du Palais Galien,
33000 Bordeaux, France

NYLANDER, G.
Department of Plastic Surgery, Hand Surgery and Burns,
University Hospital of Linköping, 85185 Linköping, Sweden

ÖHLINGER, W.
A. Ö. Krankenhaus Krems, Mitterweg 10, 3500 Krems, Austria

PALAZZI, S.
Orthopaedic and Hand Surgery Department, Centro Médico Teknon,
M. de Vilallonga, 12, 08017 Barcelona, Spain

PARISE, O.
Division of Head and Neck Surgery, Istituto Nazionale Tumori,
Via Venezian 1, 20133 Milan, Italy

PASCONE, M.
Division of Plastic Surgery, University of Trieste,
Cattinara Hospital, 34100 Trieste, Italy

PÈRES, J. M.
79, Avenue de la Marne, 64200 Biarritz, France

PESTIAUX, B.
Centre des Grands Brûlés IMTR, 6280 Loverdal, Belgium

POVLSEN, B.
Department of Plastic Surgery, Hand Surgery and Burns,
University Hospital of Linköping, 85185 Linköping, Sweden

RAMIREZ, S.
CHU Pellegrin-Tondu, Place Amélie Raba-Léon,
33000 Bordeaux, France

REDL, H.
Ludwig Boltzmann Institute for Experimental and Clinical Traumatology,
Donaueschingenstraße 13, 1200 Vienna, Austria

RIU, E.
Centro Médico Teknon, M. de Vilallonga, 12,
08017 Barcelona, Spain

RIVEL, J.
CHU Pellegrin-Tondu, Place Amélie Raba-Léon,
33000 Bordeaux, France

ROCCA, M.
Experimental Surgery, Istituto di Ricerca Codivilla Putti I.O.R.,
Via di Barbiano 1/10, 40136 Bologna, Italy

SAVANI, A.
Division of Plastic Surgery, S. Anna General Hospital,
Via Napoleona 60, 22100 Como, Italy

SCHLAG, G.
Ludwig Boltzmann Institute for Experimental and Clinical Traumatology,
Donaueschingenstraße 13, 1200 Vienna, Austria

SMAHEL, J.
Division of Hand, Plastic and Reconstructive Surgery,
Department of Surgery, University of Zürich Medical School,
8091 Zürich, Switzerland

STAINDL, O.
HNO-Abteilung der Landeskrankenanstalten Salzburg,
Müllner Hauptstraße 48, 5020 Salzburg, Austria

STARK, G. B.
Plastic and Hand Surgery Section, Universität Freiburg,
Hugstetter Straße 55, 79106 Freiburg, Germany

STERKERS, J. M.
Service d'Oto-Rhino-Laryngologie, Hôpital Beaujon,
Faculté de Médecine Xavier Bichat, Université Paris 7,
100, Bvd. Général Leclerc, 92110 Clichy, France

STERKERS, O.
Service d'Oto-Rhino-Laryngologie, Hôpital Beaujon,
Faculté de Médecine Xavier Bichat, Université Paris 7,
100, Bvd. Général Leclerc, 92110 Clichy, France

STOCKMANS, F.
Plastic and Reconstructive Surgery, University Ziekenhuizen,
Herestraat 49, 3000 Leuven, Belgium

VEDUNG, S.
Department of Plastic and Reconstructive Surgery,
University Hospital, 751 85 Uppsala, Sweden

VESIN, L.
Service des Brûlés, CHU de Tours, Hôpital Trousseau,
37044 Tours Cedex, France

VILA-TORRES, J.
Pathology Department, Centro Médico Teknon,
M. de Vilallonga, 12, 08017 Barcelona, Spain

WERBER, K. D.
Chirurgische Klinik und Poliklinik der TU München,
Klinikum Rechts der Isar, Handchirurgie,
Ismaninger Straße 22, 81664 München, Germany

WORSEG, A.
Department of Plastic and Reconstructive Surgery,
Wilhelminenspital, Montleartstraße 37, 1171 Vienna, Austria

WRIGHT, T.
University of South Alabama, Burn Center, College of Medicine,
2451 Fillingim Street, Mobile, AL 36617-2293, USA

YASSINE, A.
Service des Brûlés, CHU de Tours, Hôpital Trousseau,
37044 Tours Cedex, France

ZENG, L.
Ludwig Boltzmann Institute for Experimental and Clinical Traumatology,
Donaueschingenstraße 13, 1200 Vienna, Austria

I. Plastic Surgery

Use of Fibrin Glue in Reconstructive Plastic Surgery

T. Fabrizio, M. Nava, N. Arioli, L. Calabrese, O. Parise, R. Molinari, and A. Savani

Abstract

Human fibrin glue (Tissucol) is a plasma-derived compound endowed with adhesive and hemostatic properties and possessing a specific local anti-infection function mediated through activation of nonspecific immune elements. The aim of this randomized clinical study was to show that in patients who have undergone prolonged reconstructive plastic interventions after ablative cancer surgery following cancer resection, Tissucol decreases infectious complications. Between June 1985 and February 1992, 102 subjects were treated with fibrin glue during reconstruction operations. Analysis of the results showed that in the Tissucol group a statistically significant reduction was verified regarding both immediate complications, such as partial separation of the surgical wound and inflammation, and delayed complications, such as cicatricial hyperthrophy. In conclusion, patients treated with Tissucol showed a better quality of surgical wound, a more rapid postoperative functional recovery and, consequently, a decrease in the duration of hospitalization as compared to a control group of 112 patients.

Introduction

Fibrin seal is a compound containing a high concentration of plasma proteins such as coagulation proteins and their plasma activator. When blended, these give rise to an insoluble and stable fibrin clot, which exhibits both a hemostatic and an adhesive action combined with a biostimulating property promoting tissue repair [1–3]. A resistance to infections is achieved naturally by specific and nonspecific mechanisms since lymphocytes and antibodies as well as polymorphonuclear leukocytes (PMNs), macrophages, and plasma factors, such as complement and betalysins [4–7], are found.

The nonspecific factors come into play at a very early stage; postoperative septic complications begin in the first few hours after surgery. This is also true for depression of the reticuloendothelial system, which normally occurs after severe injury, burns, hemorrhage, and lengthy operations. The demonstration that have a precise chemotactic property, exercised by means of the fibrinogen-fibrin system, can be taken as conclusive evidence that fibrin glue possesses a

Table 1. Controlled clinical trial June 1985–February 1992: criteria for eligibility

Extensive ablations for cancer and immediate reconstructions
Negative anamnesis and laboratory tests for hepatitis B and non-A/non-B hepatitis
Informed consent

specific local anti-infection function, mediated by activation of the nonspecific immune elements. Thus, it may be concluded that in the presence of fibrin glue PMNs are mobilized in large numbers to perform their particular defensive function [8, 9].

Oncologic surgery is often characterized by extremely destructive operations which require complex reconstruction. Postoperatively, there is considerable serohematic loss. Accumulation of fluid in and around the surgical wound not only leads to flap separation and wound dehiscence, but also provides an excellent bacterical culture medium. Problems of this kind result in lengthening of the hospital stay but, much worse, may cause significant local and systemic infections [10, 11].

In order to attempt to reduce such complications, it was decided to use fibrin glue. The aim of the study was to assess the efficacy of reconstructive surgery after ablative cancer surgery. Efficacy was defined as a decrease in serohematic and infectious complications compared to a group of patients who underwent the same type of operations without the application of fibrin glue [12] (Table 1).

Material and Methods

From June 1985 to February 1992, 102 patients with various oncologic pathologies whose plastic repair involved use of human fibrin glue (Tissucol) were treated at the Istituto Nazionale Tumori in Milan (Table 2). Of these patients, 60 were male and 42 female. The age range was between 18 and 82, with an average of 50.3 years old and a median of 45 years old. Before being entered into the study, patients underwent hematology examinations testing for biohumoral hepatitis B and non-A/non-B hepatitis markers. Furthermore, each patient was subjected to the immediate hypersensitivity test by means of a subcutaneous injection of 50 μl of the Tissucol preparation, to ascertain if there was an allergic reaction. All these tests gave negative results [13, 14].

Table 2. Reconstructive plastic surgery in which fibrin glue was utilized: eligible oncological operations

Breast reconstruction with myocutaneous flaps
Head and neck reconstructions
Reconstruction of inguinal-iliac region
Composite plastic reconstructions
Reconstruction of the vulva

The total quantity of Tissucol utilized was 161.5 ml, with an average of 2.08 ml per application. The material was applied using the spray-set system; no particular postoperative antibiotic regime was performed and suction drainage was applied when indicated.

Prothombin time (PT) and partial thromboplastin time (PTT) were performed to ascertain any change in intrinsic or extrinsic coagulation which might be linked to use of human fibrin glue. These tests were performed the day before surgery, 15 days afterwards and then every 6 months.

The control group consisted of a total of 112 patients, 67 males and 45 females, whose ages ranged from 30 to 70 years, with an average age of 48 and a median of 44 years. Figure 1 illustrates the subdivision of cases in the two arms of the study by site of surgical intervention.

This study is also being conducted in the Division of Plastic Surgery, S. Anna General Hospital, Como, Italy. A total of 11 patients were recruited (Tissucol: six patients; controls: five patients), but currently their follow-up does not allow any valid conclusions.

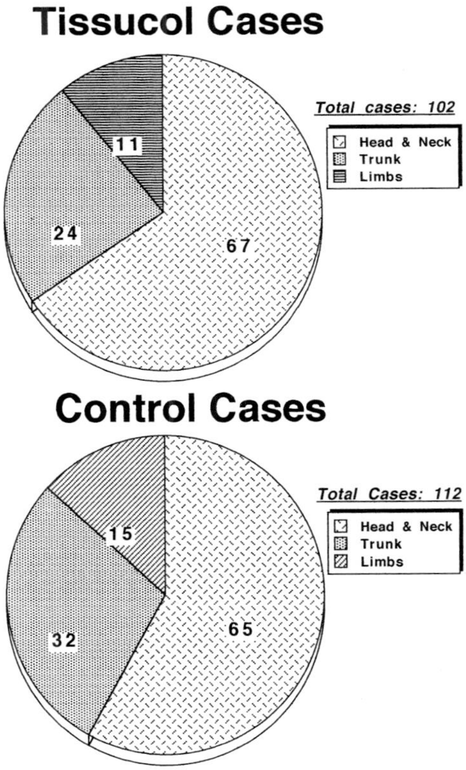

Fig. 1. Distribution of the two arms of the study according to the site of surgical operation

Results

Table 3 lists the patients treated with Tissucol and those from the control sample on the basis of the ablative and reconstructive procedures used. Resection is always followed by reconstruction, the effect of which is to produce extensive wound areas leading to considerable loss of serohematic fluid. This results in the formation of serohematic "pockets", which frequently provoke a variety of complications. This fluid is an excellent culture medium for several bacterial strains, especially gram-positive and anaerobic bacteria, which may result in wound infection, wound dehiscence, skin and fat necrosis. Additional complications are lymph collection and seromas. These complications can prolong the period of hospitalization. In our hospitals a patient with inguinal-iliac lymph node dissection requires an average postoperative hospital stay of 39 days, and wound disruption occurs in 40 %–60 % of patients.

It was decided to use Tissucol to achieve hemostasis, reduce serohematic fluid loss, seal tissues and reinforce sutures. Since Tissucol is a human plasma derivative, the possibility that viral disease such as hepatitis B or non-A/non-B hepatitis might be transmitted was evaluated. This risk can be ruled out for the following reasons: careful donor and plasma selection, product-specific heat treatment, and the clinical experience in over one million cases all over the world [15–17]. At the present time, there is no evidence of transmission of HTLV III virus in patients treated with Tissucol; also, the virus is known to be substantially unstable when exposed to heat [16, 18].

Figure 2 illustrates the main complications which can be associated with use of this product, such as those affecting coagulation, and implications resulting from the operation itself subdivided in the two arms of the study.

Hemocoagulation performed according to the study protocol consistently produced normal hematologic values, both in patients treated with Tissucol and in the control group.

Table 3. Distribution of Milan cases into the Tissucol-treated and the control groups, broken down into the type of reconstructive surgery and ablative surgery that were performed

Type of reconstruction	Type of demolition surgery	Tissucol	Controls
Head and neck reconstruction with pedicled myocutaneous flaps or free flaps	Wide demolitions and lateral cervical lymphnode dissection	67	65
Composite plastic reconstructions	Extensive ablation for malignant soft tissue tumors	20	25
Reconstruction of the inguinal-iliac with sliding cutaneous flaps	Inguinal-iliac lymphnode dissection	9	13
Breast reconstruction with latissimus dorsi myocutaneous flap	Halsted radical mastectomy	4	7
Reconstruction of the vulva with a gracilis myocutaneous flap	Total vulvectomy	2	2
Total		102	112

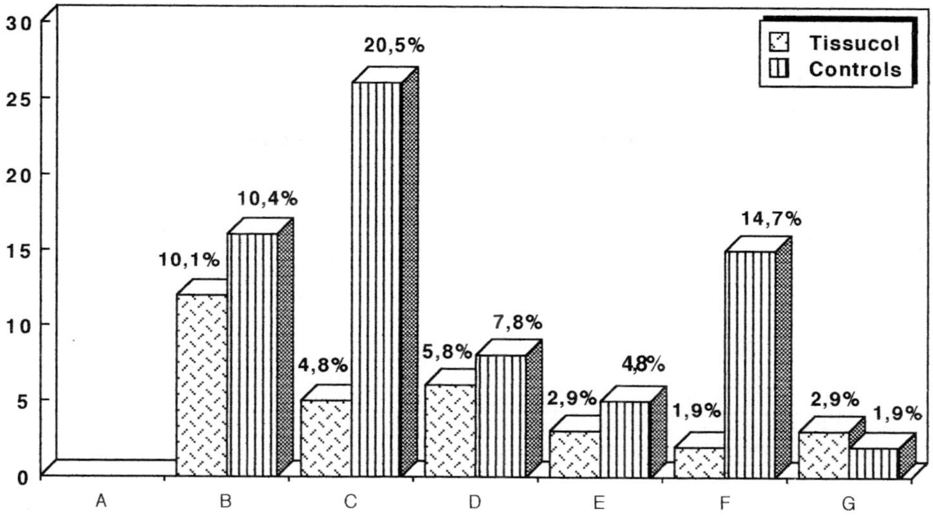

Fig. 2. Statistically relevant differences in immediate complications, such as partial separation of the surgical wound or inflammation, in the Tissucol arm vs the control arm. *A* Disorders of the intrinsic or extrinsic coagulation process; *B* serohematic fluid accumulation; *C* partial separation of the surgical wound; *D* partial necrosis of the wound; *E* hematoma; *F* inflammation; *G* lymph cysts

These data show no statistically significant differences in the incidence of seromas, lymph cysts, partial skin necrosis and hematoma between the study group and the control group. Wound dehiscence and wound inflammation show a different pattern, with a greater frequency in the control group.

Length of postoperative hospital stay ranged between 3 and 50 days for the study group, with an average of 10.5 days. In the control group the range was between 7 and 75 days, with an average of 25 days (Fig. 3).

After discharge from hospital, both groups received the same type of follow-up. A careful clinical examination to detect any delayed clinical complications was performed every 3 months during the first year following discharge, every 4 months during the second year and every 6 months from the third year on. Furthermore, every 6 months after discharge patients treated with Tissucol have undergone hematologic tests to check for the presence of the markers of hepatitis B and non-A/non-B hepatitis and to evaluate PT and PTT, checking for any coagulation disorders.

At the present stage of the follow-up, which ranges between 9 and 82 months, with an average of 44 months, tests for hepatitis B and non-A/non-B hepatitis in Tissucol treated patients have been consistently negative and the hemocoagulation values have been within the normal range.

Figure 4 illustrates the differences observed between the two groups regarding onset of delayed complications which arose during the observation period. The data show that no statistically remarkable differences can be found between the study group and the control group regarding cutaneous fistulae and lymph cysts, whereas in the onset of scar hypertrophy, statistically signifi-

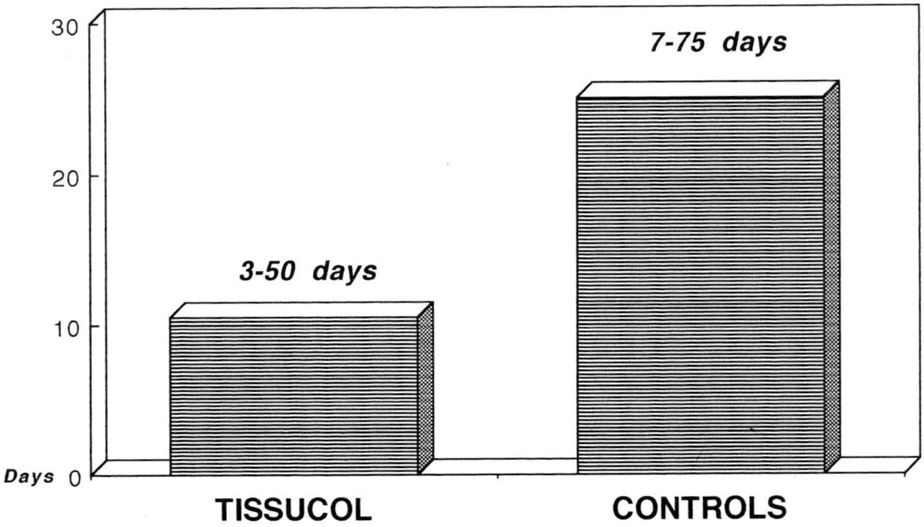

Fig. 3. Relevant differences between the Tissucol and control groups regarding post-operative hospitalization

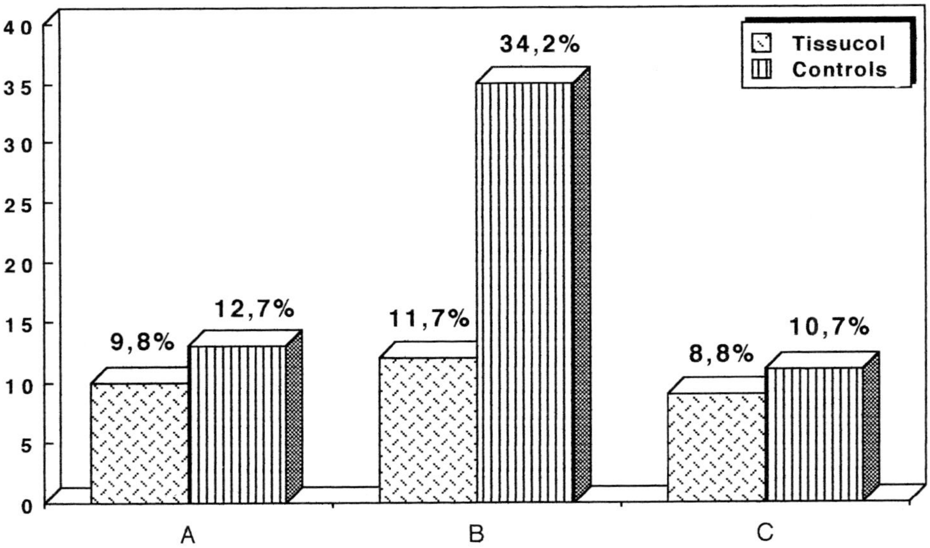

Fig. 4. Delayed complications. *A* Lymph cysts; *B* cicatricial hypertrophy; *C* cutaneous fistulae. A statistical difference was observed between the two groups for cicatricial hypertrophy

cant differences exist: 11.7% in the Tissucol group vs 34.2% in the control group.

Conclusions

The above observations on the frequency of immediate and delayed complications are consistent with a specific anti-infection function of fibrin glue, mediated through activation of PMNs. By reducing the frequency of inflammatory processes, there is a corresponding reduction in the risk of tissue inflammation and thus disruption of the surgical wound. Moreover, a decrease in the frequency of inflammation also reduces the delayed risk of hypertrophic scars.

Another favorable situation with the Tissucol group was the decrease in immediate complications, resulting in a reduction of postoperative hospital stay: 10.5 days vs 25 days in the control group. There was no substantial difference in the frequency of seromas between the two groups of patients.

Thus, Tissucol, when selectively used, reduces the frequency of onset of inflammatory processes as well as their associated immediate and delayed consequences. A better quality of surgical wound results in a more rapid postoperative functional recovery, a shorter hospital stay and therefore lower health care cost 3 (Figs. 3, 4).

Acknowledgement. Special thanks to Miss R. Parentela for her expert secretarial assistance.

References

1. Spängler HP (1976) Tissue adhesion and local hemostasis fibrinogen, thrombin and clotting factor XIII (experimental investigation-clinical experience). Wien Klin Wochenschr 88 [Suppl 49]: 3
2. Staindl O (1982) The fibrin-adhesive system in plastic surgery of head and neck. J Head Neck Pathol 3: 78
3. Staindl O (1979) The healing of wounds and scar formation under the influence of a tissue adhesion system with fibrinogen, thrombin and coagulation factor XIII. Arch Otorhinolaryngol 222: 241
4. Brandstedt S, Rank F, Olson PS (1980) Wound healing and formation of granulation tissue in normal and defibrinogenated rabbits. An experimental model and histological study. Eur Surg Res 12: 12
5. Hedelin H, Lundholm K, Teger-Nilsson AC et al. (1983) Influence of local fibrin deposition on granulation tissue formation. A biochemical study in the rat. Eur Surg Res 15: 312
6. Hunt TK, Knighton DR, Thakral KK et al. (1984) Studies on inflammation and wound healing: angiogenesis and collagen synthesis stimulated in vivo by resident and activated wound macrophages. Surgery 86: 48
7. Kasai S, Kunimoto R, Nitta K (1983) Cross-linking of fibrin by activated factor XIII stimulates attachment, morphological changes and proliferation of fibroblast. Biomed Res 4: 155
8. Donati L (1986) Indicazioni e limiti della colla di fibrina (Tissucol) in chirurgia plastica. Proceedings of the XXXVth Conference of the Italian Society of Plastic Surgery, Milan, Sept 25–27, 1986

9. Germani G (1982) Utilizzazione della colla di fibrina in chirurgia plastica. Riv Ital Chir Plast 1: 443
10. Bosh P (1980) Experimental investigation of the effect of fibrin adhesive graft. Arch Orthop Trauma Surg 96: 177
11. Cronkite EP, Lozner EL, Deaver JM (1944) Use of thrombin and fibrinogen in skin grafting. J Am Med Assoc 124: 976
12. Matras H (1982) The use of fibrin sealant in oral and maxillo-facial surgery. J Oral Maxillofac Surg 40: 617
13. Aach RD, Szmuness W, Mosley JW et al. (1981) Serum alanine aminotransferase of donors in relation to the risk of non-A, non-B hepatitis in recipients. N Engl J Med 304: 989
14. Hornbrook MC, Dood RY, Jacobs P et al. (1982) Reducing the incidence of non-A, non-B post-transfusion hepatitis by testing donor blood for alanine aminotransferase. N Engl J Med 307: 1315
15. Eder G, Neumann M, Cerwenka R, Baumgarten K (1986) Preliminary results of a randomized controlled study on the risk of hepatitis transmission of a two-component fibrin sealant in operative medicine. In: Schlag G, Redl H (eds) Traumatology – orthopaedics. Springer, Berlin Heidelberg New York, p 51 (Fibrin sealants in operative medicine, vol 7)
16. Rousou J, Gonzales-Lavin J, Cosgrove D et al. (1989) Randomized clinical trial of fibrin sealant in patients undergoing resternotomy or reoperation after cardiac operations. J Thorac Cardiovasc Surg 97: 194
17. Schricker KT, Scheele J (1981) Hepatitisrisiko der Fibrinklebung in der Allgemeinchirurgie. Med Welt 32: 783

Fibrin Sealant in Plastic Surgery of the Head

M. Pascone and D. Dioguardi

Abstract

For many years fibrin sealant has been widely used in several fields of surgery, as it has proved to be very useful in various surgical situations. The advantages offered by fibrin sealant are: (a) hemostatic effect; (b) adhesive effect; (c) biostimulating action on wound repair.

These characteristics make the use of fibrin sealant particularly useful in the treatment of congenital and acquired pathologies of the head.

In the surgery of soft tissues, the use of fibrin glue allows total adhesion of the cutaneous or myocutaneous flaps to the underlying tissues and also reduces the risk of hematomas and related infections.

Besides these advantages, Tissucol has proved to have a high degree of efficiency in surgery of the skull. It improves bone graft stability, and in skull, jaw and face injuries it can be usefully applied to fractures, especially comminuted fractures, for stabilizing small pieces of bone with a high level of accuracy.

During the past 10 years we have used fibrin sealant in many and various cases as surgical treatment including: secondary deformities resulting from injuries of the face; alveolar cleft and secondary deformities of cleft-lip-palate; cancer of the maxillofacial area; congenital deformities of the face; serious injuries of the head.

From the evaluation of clinical results, we may conclude that there are typical situations in which fibrin sealant has proven to be useful and effective.

Introduction

Based on the initial theoretical and experimental data, fibrin sealant has become a well-consolidated acquisition in the various specialized surgical fields, and by now it has many indications also in plastic surgery. As a matter of fact, over the past 10 years, several fields of Tissucol application have emerged. In some cases it is indicated as a simple, safe and rapid adhesive preparation, in others for its immediate and effective hemostatic action, and, finally, because it is able to modulate and stimulate the biological processes of tissue healing [4].

In addition Tissucol has an equally important local anti-infection function, which is mediated by activation of nonspecific immune cell elements [6].

In parallel, the remarkable advances recently achieved through surveys on bone healing biology have stirred an enormous interest regarding the clinical use of bone or bone substitute transplants. One of the outstanding indications of Tissucol consists, in fact, of bone reconstructive surgery, in which the combined use of fibrin glue with bone powder or bone fragments presents the following advantages [1, 2]: (1) precise fixation and stabilization of grafts which would be difficult with alternative means; (2) the possibility to seal sutures; this is important since bone tissue is extremely subject to infections; and (3) the possibility to fill gaps, preventing them from possible bacterial colonization.

Thanks to these characteristics, fibrin sealant has become particularly useful in treating some pathologies of the head.

Materials and Methods

This chapter describes our experience based on 70 operations, divided according to the different pathologies of the head, in which fibrin sealant was used in various ways: There were eight patients treated for consequences of trauma to the orbitomaxillofacial complex; 21 patients treated for gnathoschisis and secondary deformities; ten patients treated for maxillar and mandibular neoplasia; 18 patients treated for maxillofacial trauma; and 13 patients with congenital and acquired deformities of the head.

Consequences of Trauma of the Orbitomaxillofacial Complex

The patients belonging to this group showed an evident imbalance of the interpupillary axis, with consequent diplopia secondary to fractures of the orbitomaxillofacial complex. The latter had not been adequately treated during the acute phase because of improper evaluation or coexistence of more severe neurological problems.

In all cases treatment was carried out through transcutaneous incision of the lower lid, by repositioning the intraorbital cells and reintegrating the bone loss on the orbital floor with bone fragments (taken from tibia or iliac crest) and other tissues (lyophilized dura or temporal fascia).

Fibrin sealant was used to rapidly immobilize the tissue fragments used to fill the gaps due to bone loss on the orbital floor.

Gnathoschisis and Secondary Deformities

This group includes all patients who had bone deficiency of the alveolar process, or a deformity of the maxillae, secondary to congenital palatoschisis.

In case of gnathoschisis, our protocol consists of closure of the alveolar schisis and restoration of the continuity of the alveolar arch at about 10–11 years of age (concomitant with the appearance of the canine teeth) by using fragments of cancellous bone. The advantages include complete filling of the bone schisis; stabilization of bone stumps; raising of the ala nasi; and restoration of dental elements involved in the schisis.

The operation is carried out by preparing a mucoperiosteal pocket in the site corresponding to the schisis. The pocket is subsequently filled with cancellous bone fragments from the iliac crest and cemented together with fibrin sealant.

In patients who showed maxillary developmental deficiency consequent to labiopalatoschisis, correction of the maxillary complex has been achieved by using blocks of bovine cartilage. These were irradiated and stored in glutaraldehyde, molded, and inserted through an incision in the upper vestibular fornix, in front of the maxillary complex. Fibrin sealant was used to immobilize the cartilage blocks [3].

In all cases included in this group, fibrin sealant was also used to fill the gaps and seal the mucosal suture and make it waterproof.

Maxillary and Mandibular Neoplasia

In oncological surgery of the head, fibrin sealant was used in ten patients in whom "en bloc" removal of a cutaneous neoplasia and the underlying skeleton were carried out; in six of these patients, the lower lip and the corresponding mandibular tract were involved, while in the other four skin and bone of the orbitopalpebral region were affected.

Reconstruction of the removed skeletal segment was achieved with cortical and cancellous grafts taken from the iliac crest which were molded and fixed with metallic wire. Fibrin sealant was then used to complete hemostasis, seal the mucosal suture and promote graft healing. This was done because bone grafts or devitalized and periosteum-free grafts, as may be particularly seen in severe trauma, are likely to benefit more than other biological structures from an "early nutritional humoral intake" due to their cancellous nature.

Maxillofacial Trauma

In facial trauma, skeletal injuries can show, depending on their cause, very different clinical pictures. Although displacement of whole bone segments with considerable alterations in face structure undoubtedly represents serious reconstructive problems, the major difficulties are encountered in patients with comminuted fractures or small devascularized and periosteum-free fragments. In these cases, when normal stabilization systems are less easily usable, Tissucol is highly indicated due to its adhesive and biostimulating properties [2, 3, 7].

Congenital and Acquired Deformities of the Head

In case of deformity of the head, either congenital or secondary to trauma or surgery, Tissucol has been used to immobilize, in a simple and rapid way, fragments of autologous bone, lyophilized bovine cartilage or hydroxyapatite granules on the bone defect [5].

Results

Due to the experience we have acquired over the past 10 years, we can affirm that fibrin sealant is indicated wherever it is necessary for surgeons to have something to sustain, to amalgamate or to fill. In every application, fibrin sealant was used to immobilize fragments of bone or of other materials, to fill gaps or to staunch bleeding.

All patients experienced rapid healing, with no complication. This is of particular interest especially in surgery of the head. In fact, considering the variability and complexity of this branch of surgery, the fibrin sealant Tissucol, due to its adhesive and hemostatic properties and its stimulation of the healing process, has proved to be very useful. In traumatology, fracture bone segments are more easily stabilized, protected from infection and more rapidly integrated. When Tissucol has been used to seal bone fragments, such as in the treatment of gnathoschisis or in case of deformities or in reconstructive procedures after bone resections for tumors, X-ray follow-up, carried out some time later, showed a more rapid healing and osteogenetic process.

Discussion

By analyzing the various cases for which we have deemed it necessary to use fibrin sealant, Tissucol can be considered as a complementary reliable system in a field in which unstable results are often encountered. The successful use of Tissucol is due to its adhesive and hemostatic properties, and its ability to stimulate the healing process [10].

Even if Tissucol does not always represent an alternative method to the usual fixation and bone amalgamation techniques, this preparation is nonetheless very useful and efficacious in many surgical procedures, especially because it allows a rapid and immediate solution [8, 9].

Indeed, it is in complex biological fields, such as bone healing, that Tissucol represents an "efficacious integrative system" to be combined with bone reconstructive surgery.

References

1. Azzolini A et al. (1986) Il Tissucol in chirurgia plastica: principali applicazioni cliniche. Minerva Chir 41: 1025
2. Curioni C, Toscano P (1983) L'impiego del Tissucol in chirurgia maxillo-facciale: considerazioni su una casistica riguardante malformazioni congenite, lesioni traumatiche e neoformazioni cranio-maxillo-facciale. In: Atti del Convegno Multidisciplinare sul Tissucol, Pisa 3–5 Nov 1983
3. Dioguardi D, Pascone M, De Robertis M (1986) Utilizzazione del Tissucol nella chirurgia ricostruttiva dell'estremo cefalico. In: 35th Meeting of the National Congress of the Italian Society for Plastic Surgery, Milan 25–27 Sept 1986
4. Donati L (1986) Indicazioni e limiti della colla di fibrina (Tissucol) in chirurgia plastica. In: 35th Meeting of the National Congress of the Italian Society for Plastic Surgery, Milan 25–27 Sept 1986
5. Ferrari Parabita G, Derada Troletti G (1983) L'impiego della colla di fibrina umana (Tissucol) in chirurgia maxillo-facciale. In: Atti del Convegno Multidisciplinare sul Tissucol, Pisa, 3–5 Nov 1983
6. Jabat-Robert J (1984) Fibronectin and wound healing. In: Meeting of the European Academy of Facial Surgery, Eaubonne, 14 May 1984
7. Micali G, Stagno D'Alcontres F (1986) Utilità della colla di fibrina in chirurgia plastica. In: 35th Meeting of the National Congress of the Italian Society for Plastic Surgery, Milan 25–27 Sept 1986
8. Pascone M, De Robertis M, Giudice G, Minervini C (1985) Utilizzazione della colla di fibrina (Tissucol) in chirurgia ricostruttiva. In: 35th Meeting of the National Congress of the Italian Society for Plastic Surgery, Bari, Oct 1985
9. Scuderi N, Sposato G, Ruiz S, D'Andrea F (1986) La nostra esperienza nell'utilizzazione della colla di fibrina in chirurgia plastica. In: 35th Meeting of the National Congress of the Italian Society for Plastic Surgery, Milan 25–27 Sept 1986
10. Staindl O (1982) The fibrin-adhesive system in plastic surgery of head and neck. J Head Neck Pathol 3: 78–85

The Use of Fibrin Glue in the Operative Therapy of Dupuytren's Disease

K. D. WERBER and C. HIRGSTETTER

Abstract

The purpose of this study was to determine the usefulness of fibrin glue infiltration for prevention of hematoma formation in patients treated surgically for Dupuytren's disease. It was thought that by improving wound adhesion, better wound healing and early motion would be encountered.

Fifty patients with Dupuytren's disease underwent surgical treatment on an outpatient basis using fibrin glue in the palm. All procedures were done under axillary block using a tourniquet. Prior to tourniquet release, the skin was closed, the wound was infiltrated with 0.5 ml of fibrin glue and compression was held for 8 min, after which the dressing was applied. In only one patient did wound problems occur secondary to hematoma formation. Normal or improved wound healing occurred in all other patients with no hematoma formation.

Introduction

Based on our experience with the use of fibrin sealing at our facility as well as the work of Eide [2], we began an investigation on the use of fibrin glue in the operative treatment of Dupuytren's disease. The aim of our study was to prevent hematoma formation in the palm, one of the most feared complications of Dupuytren's disease. In achieving this, we thought better wound healing and improved early motion would result.

Materials and Methods

Partial fasciectomy was performed on 50 patients with Dupuytren's disease in an outpatient setting. All surgeries were performed under loupe magnification with careful attention to hand surgery principles [1, 3, 5, 7]. Following partial fasciectomy, hemostasis was carefully obtained. The wound was then closed over a catheter with interrupted sutures using Z-plasties when necessary (Fig. 1). Fibrin glue (0.5 ml) was then injected through the catheter using the Tissomat and compression held on the wound for 8 min (Figs. 2, 3). One end of

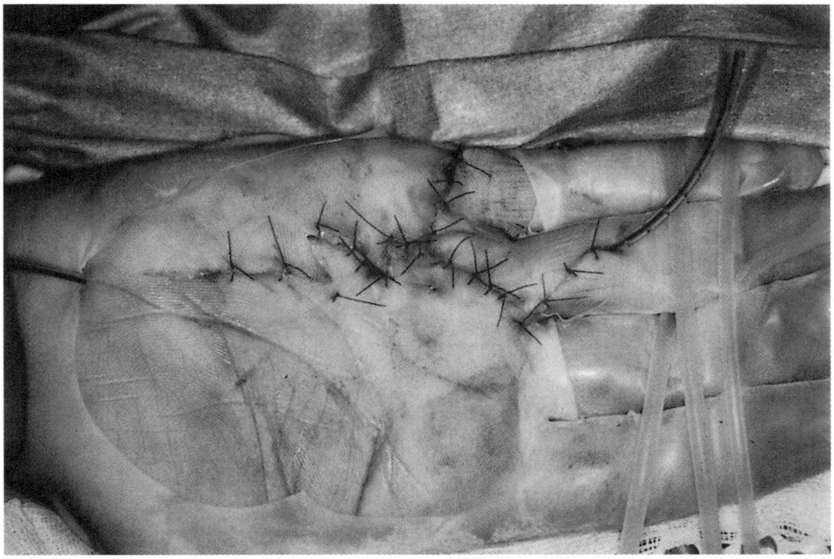

Fig. 1. Wound closure after partial fasciectomy; drain can be seen

the catheter was left in the wound to provide drainage and the tourniquet was released. The dressing was applied using a steel wool bundle to maintain light compression.

Patients were discharged from the hospital after the block had worn off and instructed to elevate the affected extremity. Discharged patients were prescribed analgesics and anti-inflammatory drugs and returned after 2 days, at which time the drain was withdrawn. The dressing was removed after 1 week, at which time therapy was initiated, and sutures were removed a week later.

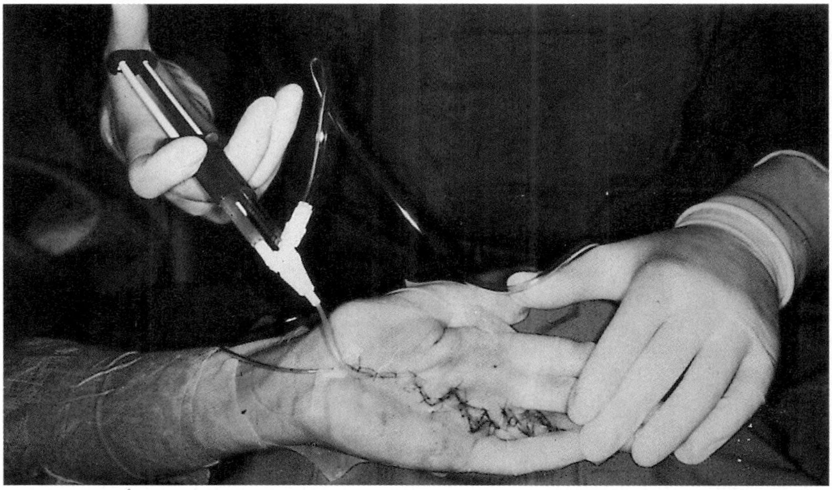

Fig. 2. Injection of Tissucol fibrin glue

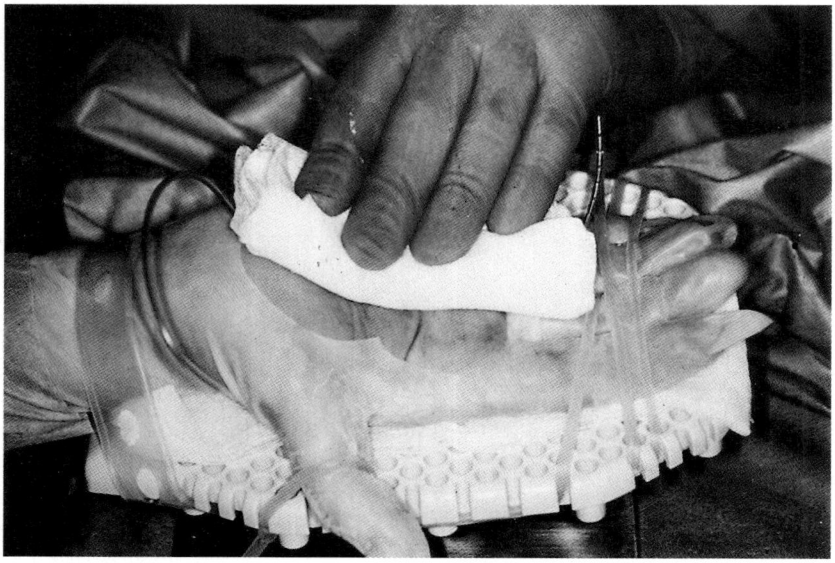

Fig. 3. Compression for 8 min

Results

Of 50 patients, hematoma occurred in only one (2 % failure rate). This was due to a technical reason (inadequate duration of compression). Three patients exhibited delayed wound healing, but did not require secondary surgery. All other patients demonstrated average or above average wound healing and better early motion.

Discussion

Hematoma formation in the palm is a serious complication following surgical treatment in Dupuytren's disease. Our purpose was to reduce the incidence of hematoma formation using fibrin glue. Hueston [4] reported a 7.5 % incidence of hematoma formation in partial and total fasciectomies. Zachariae [8] found a 17 % incidence of hematoma following partial fasciectomy and a 22.8 % incidence after total fasciectomy. Millesi [6] found rates of 4.35 % and 4.8 % for partial and total fasciectomies, respectively. Our investigation using fibrin glue revealed a decrease (to 2 %) in the rate of hematoma formation.

Conclusion

The use of fibrin glue in the operative treatment of Dupuytren's disease provides a save and effective means of hemostasis, improved wound healing and better early range of motion. Additional benefits include shorter operative time in terms of cost-benefit analysis. The fibrin glue and wound compression provide a mechanism for improved skin adhesion and elimination of dead space following wound closure.

To determine the effects of compression alone vs compression with fibrin glue, further randomized studies will be performed in the near future.

References

1. Bunnell S (1944) Surgery of the hand. Lippincott, Philadelphia
2. Eide E, Jurgeit H (1985) Die Anwendung des Fibrinklebers bei der ausgeprägten Dupuytren'schen Kontraktur. Handchirurgie 17: 145–146
3. Geldmacher J (1970) Dupuytren'sche Kontraktur. 8. Symposium der Deutschsprachigen Arbeitsgemeinschaft für Handchirurgie Vienna, May 1967. Handchirurgie [Suppl 1]: 10
4. Hueston JT (1963) Dupuytren's contracture. Livingstone, Edinburgh
5. Iselin M (1955) Chirurgie de la main. Paris
6. Millesi H (1965) Zur Pathogenese und Therapie der Dupuytren'schen Kontraktur. Eine Studie an Hand von mehr als 500 Fällen. Ergeb Chir Orthop 47
7. Skoog T (1963) The pathogenesis and etiology of Dupuytren's contracture. Plast Reconstr Surg 31: 258
8. Zachariae L (1967) Extensive versus limited fasciectomy for Dupuytren's contracture. Scand J Plast Reconstr Surg 1: 150

Osteocartilagenous Reconstruction

J. L. Eberlin, W. Hu, J. M. Pères, S. Ramirez, X. Noël, B. Basse-Catalinat, J. Rivel, and J. Baudet

Abstract

The authors drew their inspiration from the suggestions of Aebi et al. [1], at the 1987 Basel symposium, to combine several biomaterials together in order to provide an environment in which osteocartilagenous cells can differentiate and develop [2–4]. It is thus possible to get cortical, medullary or cartilagenous tissue, according to the demands of the environment, and to reconstruct a complex bone structure which is adapted to the required function [5].

Materials and Methods

The animal experiments were done on 21 young female adult rabbits (Bleu de Bourgogne) each weighing approximately 2.5 kg. The experiment consists of replacing one part of the femur by a graft of collagen glue. The diaphysis resection involved 25 % of the femoral brace and removes the periosteum, the cortex and the medulla. The epiphyseal resection involved the femoral condyles, the removed volume being at least 2 ml.

The loss of substance does not occur spontaneously if it is more than 6 mm in length, as shown by Katthagen [6], and the use of a graft becomes absolutely necessary. In our experiment the length of the resection was more than 15 mm in the diaphyseal region and 10 mm in the epiphyseal region.

The combination of slow-setting fibrin glue (Tissucol) [7] and collagen standard model IX (Osteovit) [3], sterilely and extemporaneously prepared, results in a dry, 4 cm^3 block that remains rigid in the presence of blood. After cutting and positioning the structure instead of the resections, the flaccid shifted parts are replaced to allow closure of the surgical wounds. A provisional metal structure (external and internal fixation) stabilizes the regenerating site (Table 1).

Two rabbits are killed after 8 days and the graft is inspected histologically for any sign of infection or rejection. X-ray examinations are done periodically to follow up on the integration of the grafts and their calcification. Another inspection is done on an epiphysis after 3 weeks (the rabbits are killed). Three months after the operations, all the rabbits operated on in the diaphyseal region are killed. At 3 months, two rabbits undergo a bone scintigraphy, which is also done for a grafted epiphysis.

Table 1. Operation distribution in all 21 rabbits

Operation	
Femoral diaphysis	16
Internal fixation	10
Femoral epiphysis	5
External fixation	3

Two rabbits with external fixation are anesthetized and the material is removed. These animals are kept alive for one more month to test the strength of the neoarticulation. The weight of the animals at this point is about 4 kg.

An osteodensitometric test is done on two femoral braces. All the femoral sites are examined histologically either trichromatically or with hematoxylin and eosin [5].

Results

Eight days after the operation, an influx of blood into the grafted structure can be seen histologically (Fig. 1). Pieces of various sizes of collagen are visible on a background of blood. No cellular immune reaction is visible [8].

Some 21 days after the operation, the epiphyseal graft shows a laminated surface facing the synovial fluid whereas the inside of the graft is colonized by cells of the chondroblastal type and adherence to the bone is clear.

At 3 months after the operation, bone scintigraphy shows hyperactivity in the region of the joints of the left knee where the condyles were replaced by a

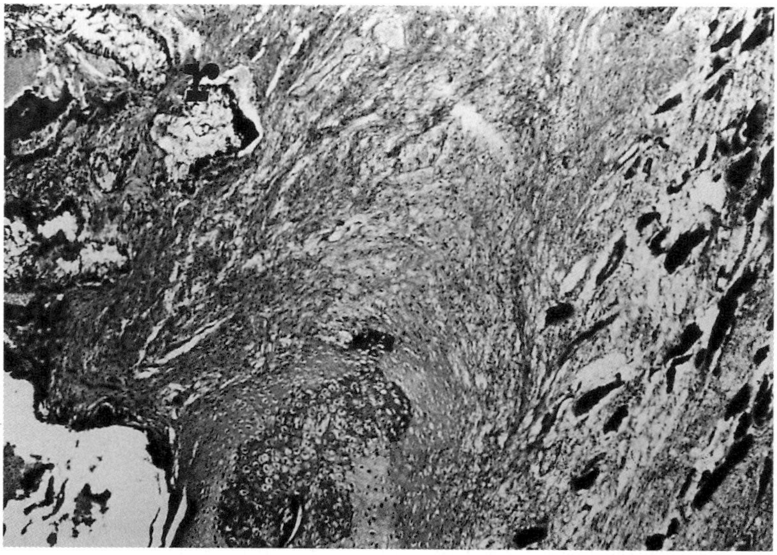

Fig. 1. Histological evaluation on day 8 shows the influx of blood into the graft without an immune reaction: *r*, structural collagen residue. Hematoxylin-eosin, × 25

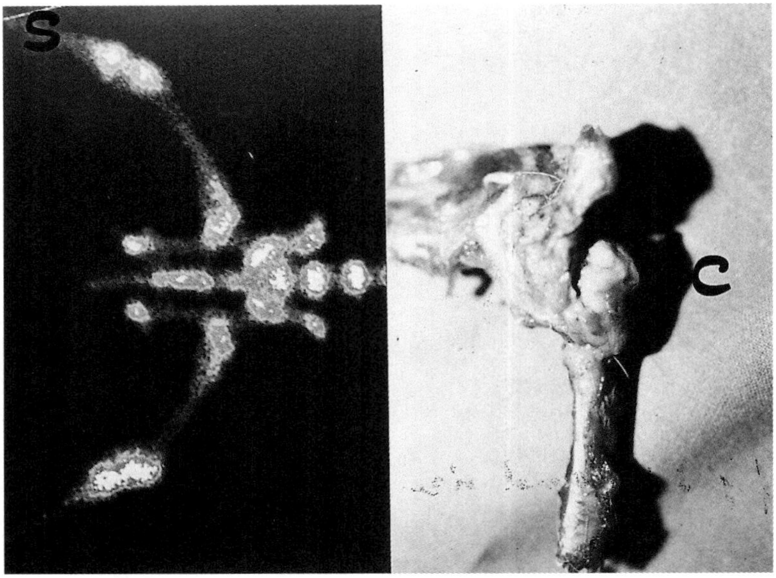

Fig. 2. Scintigraphy *(left)* in the third month shows hyperactivity of the femoral condyles and of the tibial plate. The opened knee shows the new femoral external condyle *(right)*, which is smooth, cartilagenous and homogeneous

graft. When the articular part is opened and we note cartilaginous resurfacing of the grafted part (Fig. 2).

In the diaphyseal region, after decalcification, a femoral brace is opened lengthwise which allows us to see the continuity of the structure (Fig. 3) [9–11].

The histological tests show an inrush of mature cells into the graft, either chondrocytes or osteocytes, and the beginning of a bone structure with Haversian canals (Fig. 4) [12].

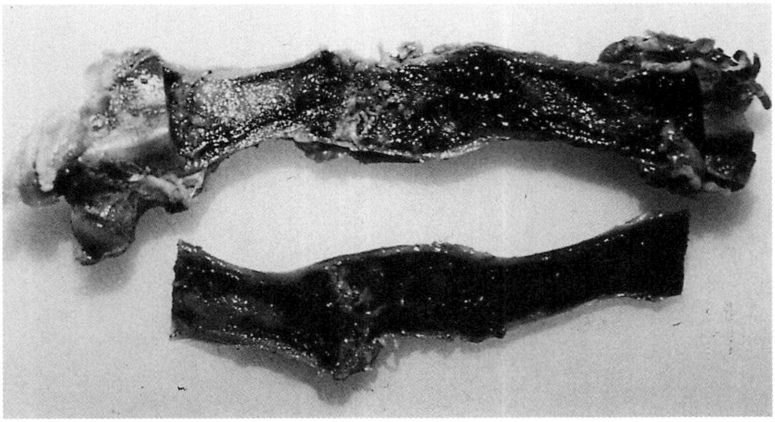

Fig. 3. The decalcified femur is cut lengthwise to show the continuity of the cortical bone and the medulla

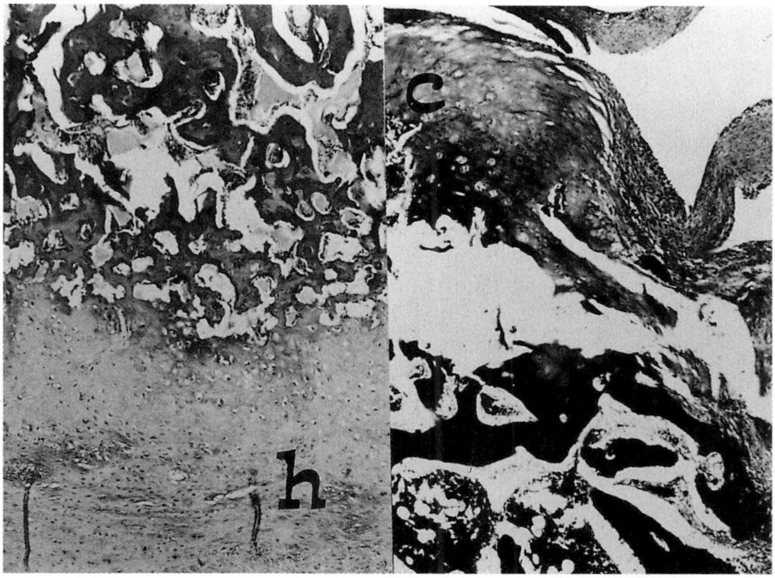

Fig. 4. Fourth month. *Left*, diaphysis stained with hematoxylin-eosin (× 100). In the grafted portion, the Haversian system is developing *(h)*. *Right*, epiphysis stained with trichrome dye, revealing the cartilagenous surface with mature chondrocytes *(c)*

Discussion

In his conclusions and as guidelines for the future of research into bone reconstruction, Aebi [1] had three main suggestions: (1) the need for a stable and mechanically viable internal structure; (2) immediate vascularization of the structure to improve the bone's chances of survival, especially for subchondral bone and cartilage; (3) the absence of any immunological reaction.

Our study addresses the third point first. One week after having operated, grafts that were removed from the rabbits showed no histological signs of immune reaction. There was no sign of inflammation and no significant concentration of leukocytes. An influx of erythrocytes provided evidence of complete vascularization of the graft.

The histology test at day 21 showed the presence of chondroblasts in the graft. This means that the bone cells of the receiving part of the femur are responding to the surrounding structures and differentiating according to the local needs, i.e., into blasts, then into osteoblasts and chondroblasts, and then maturing into osteocytes and chondrocytes. This was confirmed histologically.

The proposed graft is easy to handle and its colonization is guaranteed by the fact that the blast cells are together in a structural "desert". In particular, calcium, which acts as a structural barrier of the cortex, is absent and thus does not restrain the local influx of cells. This absence also leads to a redimensioning of the support when it comes to providing a cartilagenous structure. The receptive articular surface is thus not abraded by spicules of hydroxyapatite and remains untouched.

Conclusion

Today it is possible to propose a compound of biomaterials meeting the specifications necessary for bone reconstruction. A frame work is provided to the bone cells where they can differentiate in response to the environment and fill the existing gap [13, 14].

Acknowledgement. Our sincere thanks to Mrs. Daumy and her collaborators at the Bordeaux II research laboratory and to Dr. Bagot d'Arc, without whom this study could not have been done.

References

1. Aebi M et al. (1989) Bone transplantation-future directions in research: outlook. Springer, Berlin Heidelberg New York, pp 351–355
2. Armitage JO (1989) Bone marrow transplantation in the treatment of patients with lymphoma. Blood 73 (7): 1749–1758
3. Beckers H (1986) Möglichkeiten der Auffütterung von Weichteildefekten mit Kollagenmatrix. In: Neubauer H (ed) Plastische und Wiederherstellungschirurgie des Alters. Indikationen und Kontraindikationen. Springer, Berlin Heidelberg New York, pp 233–242 (Jahrestagung der Deutschen Gesellschaft für Plastische und Wiederherstellungschirurgie, vol 23)
4. Burchardt H (1989) Biology of cortical bone graft incorporation, bone transplantation. Springer, Berlin Heidelberg New York, pp 23–28
5. Charrier P (1981) Etude de biomatériaux utilisables en chirurgie orthopédique et réparatrice: structure et chimie du squelette madréporaire implanté dans les os de chiens. Leur résorption et la néoformation osseuse. Rapport d'étude pour le CNEXO-Hôpital R. Poincaré
6. Katthagen BD (1986) Bone regeneration with bone substitutes, an animal study. Springer, Berlin Heidelberg New York, p 143
7. Seelich T (1982) Tissucol: biochemistry and methods of application. J Head Neck Pathol 3: 65–69
8. Elves MW (1978) Cell mediated immunity to allografts and treated bone. Int Orthop 2: 171
9. Evans FG (1974) Mechanical properties of bone. Thomas, Springfield
10. Ferrari Parabita G et al. (1986) New methods of fibrin sealant application in maxillofacial surgery: the use of hydroxyapatite in association with human fibrin glue in reconstructive surgery. Plast Surg Maxillofac Dent Surg 4: 141–145
11. Harvey M Rosen, Porous (1989) Block hydroxyapatite as an interpositional bone graft substitute in orthognathic surgery. Plast Reconst Surg 83 (6): 985–990
12. Mittelmeier T et al. (1983) Klinische Erfahrungen mit Collagen-Apatit. Implantation zur lokalen Knochenregeneration. Z Orthop 121: 115
13. Romana MC et al. (1990) Vascularized periosteum associated with cancellous bone graft: an experimental study. Plast Reconst Surg 85 (4): 587–592
14. Weber M (1985) Tierexperimentelle Untersuchungen zur Knochenregeneration mit gereinigtem, xenogenem Faserkollagen und Apatitpulver. Inaugural dissertation, University of Homburg

Fibrin Sealing of Facial Skin Plasties in Older Patients

H. A. Gitt

Abstract

The number of cases of facial skin tumors in older patients calls more and more for reconstructive operations in this age group. The delayed healing and more frequent hematoma formation may jeopardize the result. With fibrin sealing it is possible to avoid the age-associated risks. Used as an adjuvant to sutures, fibrin sealing guarantees prophylaxis of hematomas and edemas, which can be dangerous for grafts and plasties. In skin plasties, fibrin sealing is applied by a simultaneous technique. Furthermore, fibrin sealing (Tisseel or Tissucol Duo S) has demonstrated its value as an adjuvant in wound surface sealing. In addition to its hemostyptic effect, we observed accelerated healing.

Introduction

For 15 years we have operated using different tissue adhesives, at first in the Maxillofacial Surgery Department and later in the Dermatosurgical Department of the University of Leipzig. First, there were various cyanoacrylates, then gelatin-resorcinol-formalin (GRF) adhesive and finally, starting in 1981, fibrin sealing (Immuno AG, Vienna). In the application of fibrin sealing two effects were generally noticed: (1) the prominent hemostyptic effect, which, especially in patients with hemorrhagic diatheses, minimized the treatment risk, and (2) the acceleration of undisturbed wound healing [2].

Of the increasing number of facial skin tumors, basal cell carcinomas have a dominating place in older patients (Figs. 1, 2). This particular risk group places high demands on the dermatosurgeon with regard to plastic-reconstructive methods, especially in the facial region [1, 3, 4, 6]. Age-induced caused physiological alterations, above all in the vessels, allow formation of hematomas and/or edemas more frequently than in younger patients. This is dangerous for the skin plasties [7].

Beside general conditions caused by old age, accompanying diseases, e.g. diabetes, delay or endanger wound healing or healing of the skin plasties [5, 8].

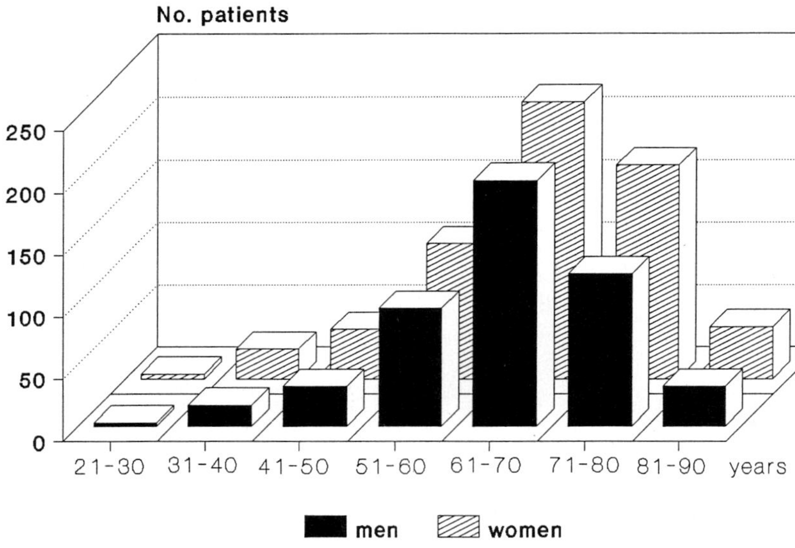

Fig. 1. Age distribution in basal cell carcinoma patients 1967–1971

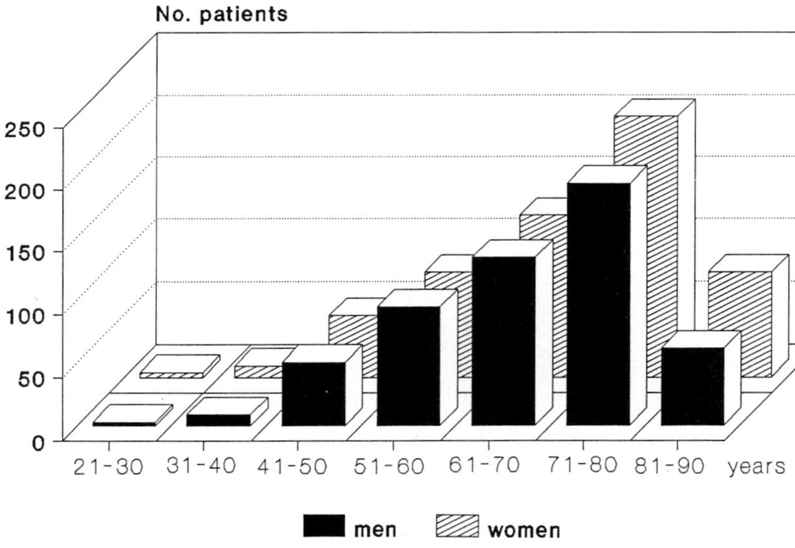

Fig. 2. Age distribution in basal cell carcinoma patients 1982–1986

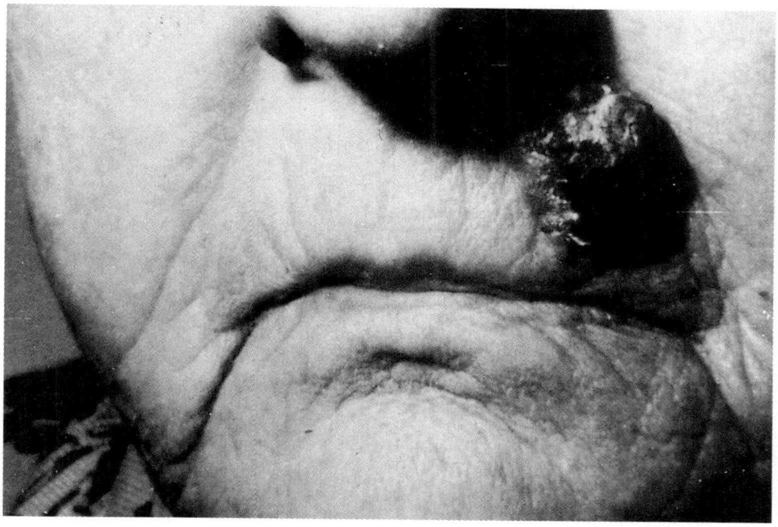

Fig. 3. Surgical treatment of basal cell carcinoma (female, 82 years)

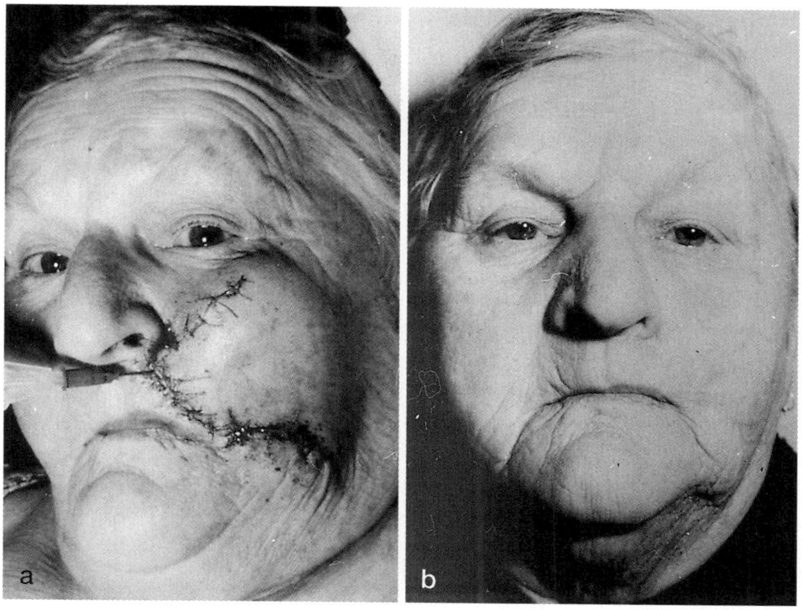

Fig. 4a, b. Flap operation **a** after tumor excision and Tisseel application; **b** final result after 8 weeks

Table 1. Patients treated with fibrin sealing (October 1992)

Number of patients	237
Sex	125 males 112 females
Age (average)	77.3 years
Minimum	58.2 years
Maximum	97.1 years

Material and Methods

Based on our preliminary experience, we applied fibrin sealing in 237 patients (Table 1). In 173 patients who underwent plastic surgery we used pedicled flaps for reconstruction after tumor surgery (Figs. 4, 5). In 52 patients we used grafts (skin grafts or composite grafts). In 12 patients we used the method in treatment of rhinophymas or nevi following dermabrasions:

1. We operate preferably with the Tisseel Kit, because we can control the speed of polymerization. The advantages are that we can use the time before onset of polymerization to adapt the graft.
2. We prefer nearly exclusively the simultaneous application technique, to guarantee that in the whole operation field the mixture of both components is exactly the same.
3. Fibrin sealing is mostly used as an adjuvant to sutures and in minimizing the number of sutures. The exception is spray application after dermabrasion of greater nevi or in the treatment of rhinophymas.

Results

The successful application of fibrin sealing in facial skin plasties in older patients supports plastic-reconstructive operations in this group. The operation time can be shortened, since fewer sutures are required and hemostasis is reliable. In more than 200 patients, an exact intraoperative hemostasis was provided. We found that by using fibrin sealing, the formation of hematomas and edemas was less frequent than without fibrin sealing. Wound healing and healing of skin plasties can proceed undisturbed, since there are no hematomas and fewer infections. Moreover, the healing time is shorter (on average 3–5 days), as compared to plasties without Tisseel which take up to 10 days to heal. The aesthetic results are very satisfactory, since wounds heal better and more quickly. The high cost is balanced by the shortened treatment time.

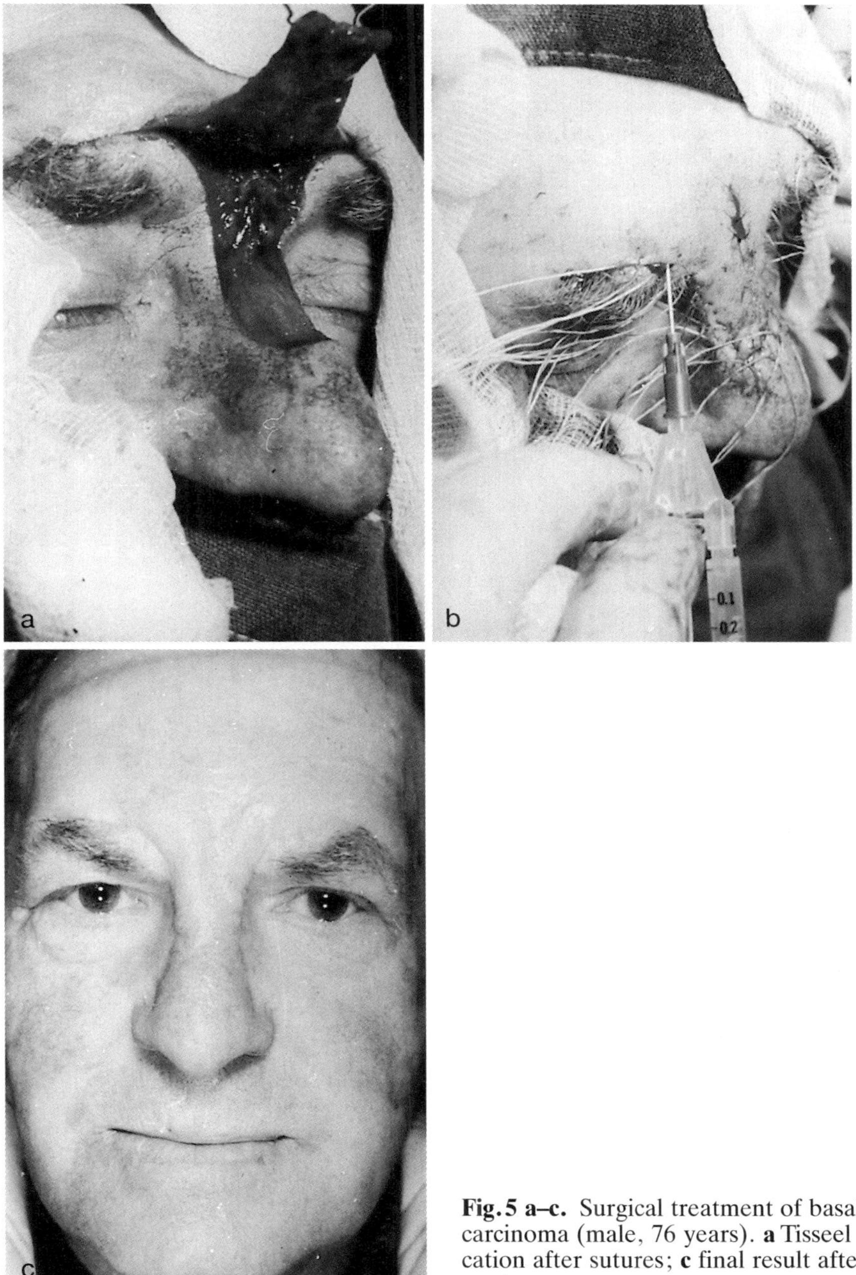

Fig. 5 a–c. Surgical treatment of basal cell carcinoma (male, 76 years). **a** Tisseel application after sutures; **c** final result after 4 weeks

References

1. Drommer RB, Hotz G (1991) Fibrinklebung in der Mund-, Zahn- und Kieferheilkunde. Springer, Berlin Heidelberg New York
2. Gitt HA, Bethmann W (1986) The use of fibrin sealant in various maxillosurgical indications. In: Schlag G, Redl H (eds) Plastic surgery – maxillofacial and dental surgery. Springer, Berlin Heidelberg New York, p 152 (Fibrin sealant in operative medicine, Vol 4)
3. Mang WL (1988) Fibrinklebung in der ästhetischen Gesichtschirurgie: ein Fortschritt? In: Zellner PR (ed) Fibrinklebung in der Verbrennungschirurgie – Plastischen Chirurgie. Springer, Berlin Heidelberg New York, p 66
4. Münker R (1989) Gewebeklebung in der ästhetischen Chirurgie. In: Gosepath J (ed) Aktuelle Methoden der Gewebeklebung im Kopf-Halsbereich. Urban and Schwarzenberg, Munich, p 65
5. Odar J (1990) Techniken und Methoden der modernen Medizin. Steinkopff, Darmstadt
6. Pitanguy J (1981) Esthetic plastic surgery of head and body. Springer, Berlin Heidelberg New York
7. Sohn SA, Sheen JH (1987) Fundamentals of aesthetic plastic surgery. Williams and Wilkins, Baltimore
8. Staindl O (1988) Fibrinklebung bei plastischen Operationen im Kopf- und Halsbereich. In: Zellner PR (ed) Fibrinklebung in der Verbrennungschirurgie – Plastischen Chirurgie. Springer, Berlin Heidelberg New York, p 62

Hemangioma Treatment with Fibrin Sealant

A. Krüger

Abstract

Since 1980, more than 100 patients have been treated for cavernous and capillary hemangiomas using fibrin sealant and magnesium thread. Excellent results can be achieved by forming a thrombosis following injection of sealant into the hemangioma.

With infants and small children, fibrin sealant and magnesium thread implant is injected directly into the vessel convolution after a computed tomography image has been made. Thrombosis of the hemangioma is followed by fibrosis, until the hemangioma gradually wastes away. Thus an operation can be avoided. The treatment can be performed several times.

In adults, fibrin sealant and a magnesium thread implant are performed once and, after thrombosis, complete extirpation of the whole hemangioma can easily be carried out.

Histological investigations showed fibrosis and sclerosis of granulated tissue enriched with fibroblasts. No sign of inflammation could be observed.

Patients are treated in our office facilities. There is no risk of emboli and can easily be managed by the medical staff.

Introduction

I have been using the technique of fibrin sealant injection since 1980 and I would like to thank Prof. Otto Staindl from Salzburg – whose excellent results are well known – for his inspiring presentation in Berlin. Since the Berlin symposium I have been following his advice, additionally injecting 99 % magnesium thread together with fibrin sealant. This seems to be a forgotten method. It was originally established by von Payr in 1900 and brings about a stronger fibrosis of cavernous hemangiomas.

The advantage of combining both techniques in newborn and small children lies in the involution of the frequently growing hemangiomas. Thus we can postpone surgery until the patient reaches adolescence.

In adult patients a magnesium implantation and fibrin sealant injection can provoke a significant reduction of the hemangioma and thus – due to the thrombosis – provides a change to operate on the hemangioma without any risk of recurrence.

Material and Methods

In addition to cryosurgical icing with liquid nitrogen dioxide, injection of fibrin sealant – used earlier in combination with magnesium implantation – has proved highly effective. For the treatment of superficial hemangiomas laser therapy must also be considered.

Prophylaxis

The need to inform pediatricians and gynecologists about small hemangiomas in newborns should be strongly emphasized in order to arrange necessary treatment.

In the case of an 11-months-old baby, this treatment opportunity was missed. The child is now going to be treated with fibrin and magnesium injections. Another child was radiologically examined by computed tomography – a standard measure to exclude further hemangiomas, especially at the skull-base – prior to the injection. Some 4 weeks later, a distinct involution could be observed.

The self-healing potential of hemangiomas, which becomes effective in 90 % of all cases, is activated in the other 10 % by the fibrin injection.

The first child treated by us in 1980 had a good result and involution of the hemangioma. The child is now 13 years old and has never undergone an operation, except for a histologic puncture.

Results

Complications

In far more than 100 cases of fibrin sealant injections in treating hemangiomas, we have not observed any side effects or risks. In all case studies we documented a major reduction of the hemangioma by fibrosis. However, one patient showed a special complication: the injection of 3 ml of sealant into a large cheek hemangioma of an adult caused a shock reaction similar to allergic anaphylaxis. It was handled and solved by well-known emergency methods. Later on, the same patient received further injections without any complications.

Blood analysis following the injection of fibrin sealant showed an increase of fibropeptides in the patients. Therefore, theoretically one has to consider an increased risk of embolism. For these investigations, a pool of only ten patients was available. Thus, our final results are of only relative validity. Nevertheless, we did not observe any sign of embolism in our more than hundred case studies.

Case Studies

One child with a hemangioma of the upper eyelid and the brow was treated several times befor we could perform extirpation of the remaining hemangioma. Another child was operated on for hemangioma without any problems after an injection therapy of 2 years. A child with a huge hemangioma of the upper lip was treated with repeated injections. An operation has thus been avoided so far.

Finally, there was a case of a patient with a hemangioma of the external ear. Due to frequent bleeding, the patient had to be operated on 12 times, whereas only one injection of Tissucol improved the result significantly.

As to the technique of injection I would like to emphasize that, during and after the injection, a 3 min compression of the surrounding tissue must be strictly observed.

Suggested Reading

1. Bell J (1826) Principles of surgery. In: Bell C (ed) On the aneurysma per anastomosin, vol 3. Frouriep, Weimar
2. Dennecke HJ, Hartert H (1954) Carotis-Interna-Verletzungen mit unstillbarem Nasenbluten, geheilt durch intraarterielle Thrombin-Injektionen. Chirurg 25: 470–472
3. Hundeiker M (1978) Systematik der vaskulären Neubildungen. Hautarzt 29: 565–572
4. Hundeiker M (1985) Fehlbildungen des Gefäßsystems, Systematik. In: Wolff HH, Schmeller W (eds) Fehlbildungen, Naevi, Melanome. Springer, Berlin Heidelberg New York, pp 32–41
5. Krüger A (1985) Neue Aspekte zur Haemangiom-Behandlung. HNO 33: 498–492
6. Lexer E (1918) Lehrbuch der allgemeinen Chirurgie, vol 2. Enke, Stuttgart, pp 292–300
7. Payr E (1902) Über Verwendung von Magnesium zur Behandlung von Blutgefäßerkrankungen. Dtsch Z Chir 63: 503
8. Payr E (1900) Beiträge zur Technik der Blutgefäß- und Nervennaht nebst Mitteilungen über die Verwendung des resorbierenden Metalles in der Chirurgie. Arch Klin Chir 62: 67–72
9. Payr E (1903) Zur Technik der Behandlung kavernöser Tumoren. Zentralbl Chir 47: 233–237
10. Payr E (1905) Weitere Erfahrungen über die Behandlung von Blutgefäßgeschwülsten mit Magnesiumpfeilen. Zentralbl Chir 49: 1335–1340
11. Sauerbruch (1909) Die Behandlung der Angiome mit gefrorener Kohlensäure. Zentralbl Chir 36: 1–3
12. Krüger A (1986) New aspects of haemangioma treatment. In: Schlag G, Redl H (eds) Plastic surgery – maxillofacial and dental surgery. Springer, Berlin Heidelberg New York (Fibrin sealant in operative medicine, vol 4), pp 127–132
13. Staindl O, Esca S (1984) Zur Diagnose und operativen Behandlung von Naevi und Haemangiomen im Kopf- und Halsbereich. Laryngol Rhinol Otol 63: 545–555
14. Staindl O (1989) Treatment of hemangiomas of the face with magnesium seeds. Arch Otorhinolaryngol 246: 213–217
15. Staindl O (1985) Indications of the fibrin sealant in facial plastic surgery. Fac Plast Surg 2: 323–339
16. Staindl O: Klinik und Therapie der Hämangiome. HNO 36: 259–266
17. Wallace HJ (1953) The conservative treatment of haemangiomatous naevi. Br J Plast Surg 6: 78–82

Magnesium Seeds and Fibrin Sealant for the Therapy of Hemangiomas

O. Staindl

Abstract

Various conservative and surgical procedures are available for the management of aggressive hemangiomas in infancy and childhood. One of them is magnesium seeding in combination with fibrin sealant. The technique consists of implanting 1-mm-thick wires of 99.8 % pure magnesium and fibrin sealant into the tumor mass. During repeated courses oxidation of the metal results in fibrosis and cicatricial transformation of the tumor. Indications, technique, and results are discussed.

Introduction

Hemangiomas are relatively common tumors in infancy and childhood. Depending on their size and localization, these benign neoplasms can be fraught with problems, both in terms of the need for treatment and the treatment itself. As angiomatous nevi they are true neoplasms, caused by the proliferation of endothelial cells, and predominantly affect females. Transitory dysregulation of the mechanisms controlling vascular growth is thought to be the causal factor underlying the development of the capillary masses [1]. Infantile or "strawberry" hemangiomas occur in 2 %–3 % of all infants. These tumors are initially characterized by single or multiple reddish, soft nodules of diffusely delineated spots [2]. Between 2 and 5 weeks of age, these early lesions grow rapidly to form bright-red, soft tumor masses.

While hemangiomas are characterized by rapid early growth, they tend to cease growing at about the 15th week of life and regress gradually [3]. In general, spontaneous regression follows a specific pattern: lesions lose 50 % of their volume by the age of 5 years, 70 % by age 7 years and 90 % by age 9 years. In most instances the skin changes left are cosmetically quite acceptable. As a general rule, hemangiomas can be expected to lose roughly 10 % of their volume each year [4].

Indications for Treatment

Since about 95 % of all of hemangiomas in infancy and childhood can be expected to regress spontaneously [5], initial treatment should always be "wait and see." This approach will spare many children an unnecessary or even disfiguring operation. Intervention should be reserved for hemangiomas which do not show any tendency to regress or which are likely to become complicated [6, 7].

Complications associated with hemangiomas may be local or systemic. Local complications include hemorrhages, ulcerations and arrested development of vital organs affected. Hemangiomas of the eyelids may lead to amblyopia, while those of the nose or upper lip may interfere with normal development. Masses localized in the neck may obstruct the airways, and those affecting the oral cavity may result in feeding problems. Systemic complications include Kasabach-Merritt's syndrome [8], heart failure secondary to hemodynamic impairment by the extensive vascular spaces of giant hemangiomas, and potentially life-threatening gastrointestinal hemorrhages. Additionally, lesions in adults may result in serious psychosocial problems. Facial hemangiomas may at times reach a grotesque size and cause major disfigurements. Those lesions particularly affecting the nose and the lips may result in deformities, stigmatizing patients more than any other facial lesion. All of these factors should be regarded as absolute indications for treatment.

Treatment of hemangiomas that have not regressed or those associated with complications has included corticosteroids, embolization, cryotherapy, radiotherapy and surgery (which can be limited or radical). All of these modalities have their specific indications, but they should be deferred as long as possible or until clinical circumstances require their use. A discussion of their use, however, is beyond the scope of this report.

The implantation of magnesium seeds is an old therapeutic approach. It was developed more than 90 years ago to ensure early involution of angiomas in need of treatment and has recently received renewed attention. Seeds were first implanted in a hemangioma by Nicoladoni in 1893. The method was first reported by Payr [9–12] in 1900 and continued to be used until the 1920s. It then fell into abeyance, but was rediscovered by Wilflingseder and associates [13–16] in the early 1980s.

Material and Methods

Seeds consist of 99.8 % pure magnesium (Goodfellow Metals, Cambridge, UK). The material is available by the yard at a thickness of 0.25–0.5 mm and a diameter of 1.0 mm. We prefer 1.0 mm wires because of their convenient handling. After autoclaving, 1.5–2 cm long pieces of wire are immersed in 10 % acetic acid for several seconds. In the acid bath, oxygen is released and the originally gray metal becomes bright white. The metal pieces are then rinsed and implanted either directly or through large-bore hypodermic needles serving as trocars. Depending on the size of the mass to be treated, 25–80 cm of the magnesium wires are implanted in each treatment course. Any major bleeding from puncture sites is controlled by superficially placed absorbable sutures. To prevent bleeding into tissues, fibrin sealant is injected into the mass [17]. The exclusive use of fibrin sealant (Tissucol) for useful therapy of cavernous and capillary hemangiomas was first described by Krüger 1985 [18]. He injected fibrinogen and thrombin-solution directly into the vascular convolution, resulting in complete thrombosis with subsequent fibrosis and leading to diminution of the hemangioma until it finally disappeared. In a large number of adults reduction of the tumor mass was successfully achieved, followed by immediate surgical removement of the entire tumor.

A combined magnesium-fibrin sealant therapy provides two benefits: first, the immediate sealing of bleedings after magnesium seeding and second, the enforcement of the therapeutic effect.

The efficacy of the treatment described is based on the oxidation of chemically almost 100% pure magnesium. In this process hydrogen ions are released into the tissues being treated to cause fibrosis. About 2 weeks after implantation, the magnesium wires are gradually absorbed. Depending on the thickness of the wires, absorption is complete within 8–12 weeks. Extensive experimental and clinical studies have shown the magnesium seeding to be almost entirely devoid of hazards. Irritation of adjacent connective tissues, muscles and nerves, etc. is absent [19–21] and magnesium blood levels have remained within normal limits.

Seeding can be repeated as often as is desired. Treatment is terminated once tumor involution has occurred, or it can be followed by a final surgical procedure to extirpate any residual tumor tissue. Depending on the tumor size, treatment is likely to last 1.5–2 years. In general, hemangiomas show definite paling after the very first treatment course. Reticular, whitish fibrous strands are seen to develop, and the livid, tautly elastic tumor growth turns into a somewhat firmer fibrous grayish-white mass.

Results

Histologically, untreated infantile hemangiomas in the skin are characterized by dilated capillaries with endothelial thickening in the papillary layer. Mitoses are rare. During further development the lesions extend to the reticular layer, and buds of spindle-shaped cells with longitudinal reduplication are surrounded by loose cellular connective tissue. In the subcutaneous tissue capillary buds and newly formed capillaries form networks between fat cells. In the tuberonodose variant, ectatic dilatations are more prominent than capillary proliferations. Their walls invariably show the structure of capillaries (Fig. 1).

Hemangiomas treated by magnesium seeding undergo progressive fibrosis as the seeds are absorbed. Fibrosis is characterized by the ingrowth of fibroblasts and fibrocytes. Thrombosis of the ectatic cavernous capillaries occurs with thickening of their walls and fibrous transformations. Vascular structures are gradually replaced by both loosely arranged and firm cicatricial and fibrous tissue. Muscles and neural structures are unaffected (Fig. 2). These histological

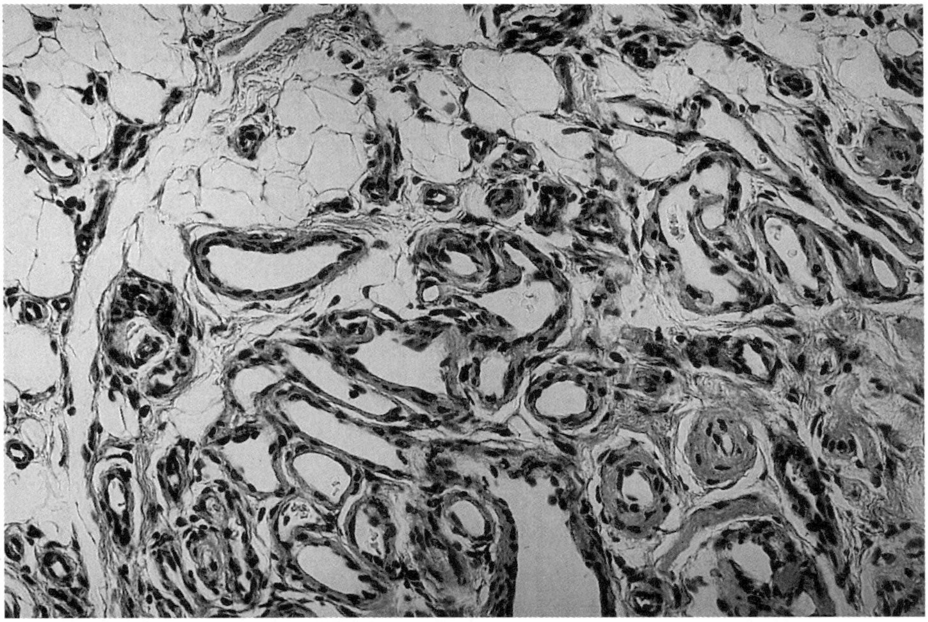

Fig. 1. Untreated hemangioma. Hematoxylin & eosin, ×45

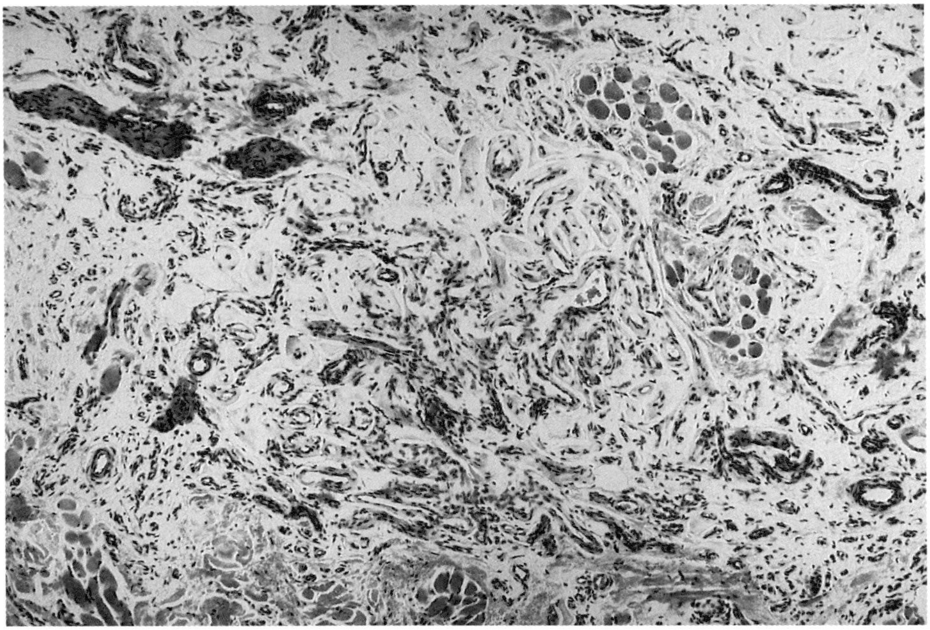

Fig. 2. Tumor histology after magnesium seeding is characterized by fibrosis, thrombosis and ingrowth of fibroblasts and fibrocytes. ×55

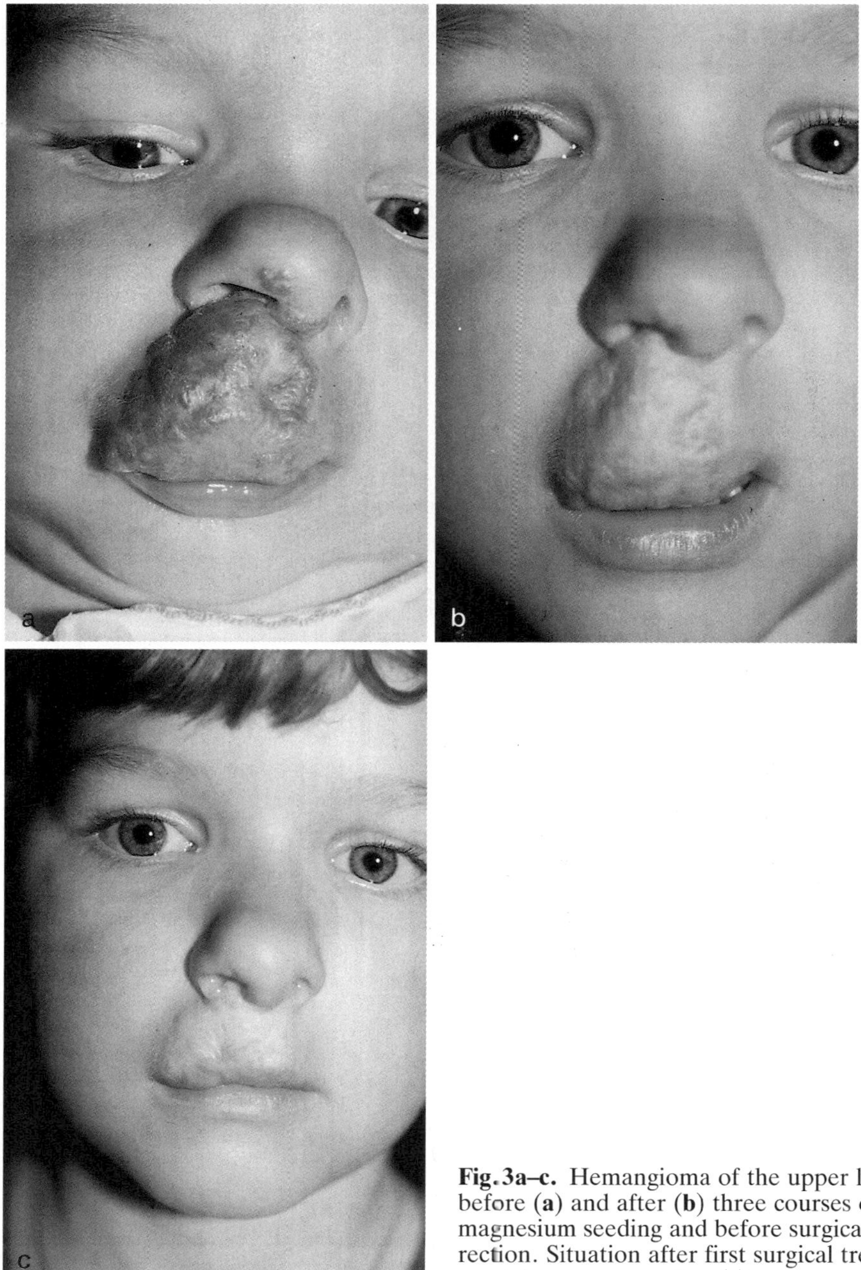

Fig. 3a–c. Hemangioma of the upper lip before (**a**) and after (**b**) three courses of magnesium seeding and before surgical correction. Situation after first surgical treatment for scar correction (**c**)

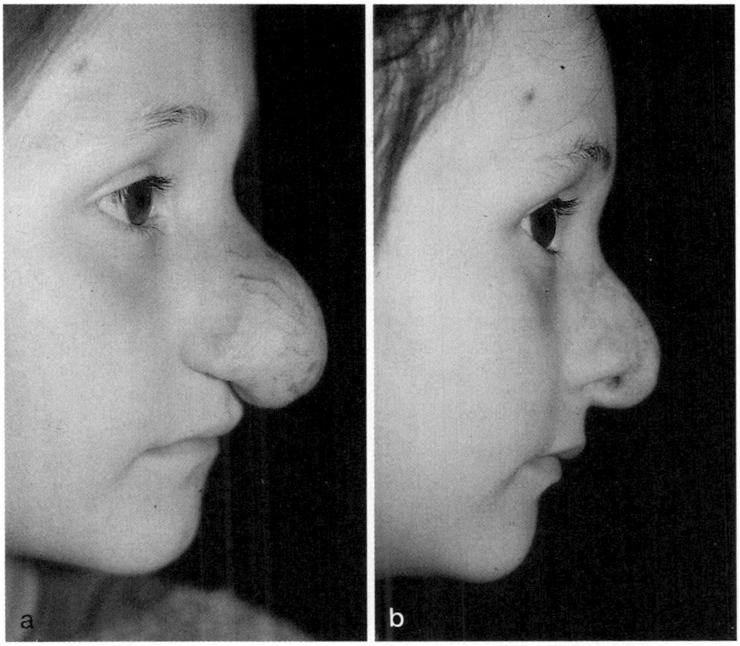

Fig. 4a, b. Excessive hemangioma of the nose before (**a**) and after (**b**) three courses of magnesium seeding

transformations are consistent with gross clinical impressions, i.e., reduction in blood volume, paling, involution and cicatricial shrinkage of the tumor mass (Figs. 3, 4).

Discussion

About 95 % of hemangiomas in childhood are known to regress spontaneously. The critical reader might, therefore, be tempted to attribute the success of magnesium seeding to the natural involutional tendency of the tumor. However, the natural history of hemangiomas is best characterized by an involution of about 10 % annually, while magnesium seeding usually produces complete involution within roughly 2 years, so that the efficacy of this treatment modality appears to be well documented [22–26].

If spontaneous involution of tumor does not occur (roughly 5 % of patients) or the measures used for magnesium seeding fail to produce complete regression, surgical extirpation is indicated. Depending on the size of the tumor, reconstructive procedures include primary closure, local flaps or free skin grafting for cosmetically satisfactory wound repair.

References

1. Hundeiker M (1978) Systematik der vaskulären Neubildungen. Hautarzt 29: 565–572
2. Hundeiker M (1985) Fehlbildungen des Gefäßsystems: Systematik. In: Wolff HH, Schmeller W (eds) Fehlbildungen, Naevi, Melanome. Springer, Berlin Heidelberg New York, pp 32–41
3. Wallace HJ (1953) The conservative treatment of hemangiomatous nevi. Br J Plast Surg 6: 78–82
4. Schnyder UW (1966) Erbliche Gefäßmäler, Teleangiektasien und Lymphödeme. In: Gottron A, Schnyder UW (eds) Handbuch der Haut- und Geschlechtskrankheiten, suppl, vol 7. Springer, Berlin Heidelberg New York, pp 695–742
5. Grothusen G (1968) Spontane Rückbildungsvorgänge an Hämangiomen des Säuglingsalters. Aesthet Med 17: 27–34
6. Drepper H, Tilkorn H, Hundeiker M (1985) Indikationen zur chirurgischen Behandlung von Hämangiomen und Angiektasen im Kindesalter. In: Wolff HH, Schmeller W (eds) Fehlbildungen, Naevi, Melanome. Springer, Berlin Heidelberg New York, pp 53–66
7. Matthews DW (1954) Treatment of haemangiomata. Br J Plast Surg 6: 83–89
8. Kasabach HH, Merritt KK (1940) Capillary haemangioma with extensive purpura. Report of a case. Am J Dis Child 59: 1063–1069
9. Payr E (1900) Beiträge zur Technik der Blutgefäß- und Nervennaht nebst Mitteilungen über die Verwendung des resorbierbaren Metalles in der Chirurgie. Arch Klin Chir 62: 67–72
10. Payr E (1902) Über die Verwendung von Magnesium zur Behandlung von Blutgefäßerkrankungen. Dtsch Z Chir 63: 903–906
11. Payr E (1903) Zur Technik der Behandlung kavernöser Tumoren. Zentralbl Chir 47: 233–237
12. Payr E (1905) Weitere Erfahrungen über die Behandlung von Blutgefäßgeschwülsten mit Magnesiumpfeilen. Zentralbl Chir 49: 1335–1340
13. Wilflingseder P (1965) Grundsätze der chirurgischen Behandlung von Hämangiomen. Klin Med 20: 245–249
14. Wilflingseder P (1967) Möglichkeiten und Grenzen der Hämangiomchirurgie. Acta Chir Plast 9: 153–156
15. Wilflingseder P, Propst A (1972) Klinische und morphologische Aspekte zur Cortison-Therapie von Hämangiomen. Chir Plast 1: 109–118
16. Wilflingseder P, Martin R, Papp C (1981) Magnesium seeds in the treatment of lymph- and haemangioma. Chir Plast 6: 105–116
17. Staindl O (1985) Indications of the fibrin sealant in facial plastic surgery. Fac Plast Surg 2: 4: 232–339
18. Krüger A (1985) Neue Aspekte zur Haemangiom-Behandlung. HNO 33: 489–492
19. Glas E (1926) Klinische und experimentelle Untersuchungen über die Payr'sche Magnesium-Behandlung. Dtsch Z Chir 194: 354–359
20. Hussl H, Papp C, Höpfel-Kreiner I, Rumpl E, Wilflingseder P (1981) Resorption time and tissue reactions with magnesium rods in rats and rabbits. Chir Plast 6: 117–126
21. Wunderer S, Strassl H (1975) Metallchirurgische Untersuchungen von Magnesium zur Spickungstherapie von Hämangiomen. Cat Chir Aust 7: 80–82
22. Staindl O (1988) Klinik und Therapie der Hämangiome. HNO 36: 259–266
23. Staindl O, Esca S (1984) Zur Diagnose und operativen Behandlung von Naevi und Haemangiomen im Kopf- und Halsbereich. Laryngol Rhinol Otol 63: 545–555
24. Staindl O (1989) Treatment of hemangiomas of the face with magnesium seeds. Arch Otorhinolaryngol 246: 213–217
25. Staindl O (1991) Hemangiomas of the lips: treatment with magnesium seeds. Fac Plast Surg 7 (2): 114–118
26. Staindl O (1992) Magnesiumspickung in der Therapie der Säuglingshaemangiome. Otorhinolaryngol Nova 2: 46–50

II. Nerve Repair

Tissucol in Peripheral Nerve Repair: An Experimental Study in the Rat

W. Boeckx, F. Stockmans, and P. Guelinckx

Abstract

This experiment was set up to compare under ideal conditions perineural nerve repair with 10-0 microsurgical sutures and fibrin adhesive perineural nerve repair. A histological and physiological evaluation was done four months postoperatively.

As model the biggest fascicle of the sciatic nerve was used. This is the fascicle for the n. tibialis posterior. In twelve male Wistar rats the biggest fascicle was dissected free from its epineurium under an operating microscope. The two other fascicles were left intact. By doing so the tension on the suture was partly avoided and the other fascicles were supported and splinted. An incision was made in the midthigh to expose the sciatic nerve. Hemostasis was performed with bipolar coagulation. The fascicle was cut using microsurgical scissors and then repaired with three stitches at 120° or with tissue adhesive. In order to have matching pairs, every animal was operated on both sites (one site with the stitches, the other with tissue adhesive). For repair with tissue adhesive one surgeon aligned the two nerve stumps with two Dumont forceps no. 5 at 25 times magnification while the other puts a drop of the fibrinogen solution followed by the thrombin solution on the aligned nerve stumps.

Four months postoperatively we physiologically evaluated the contraction properties of the innervated gastrocnemic muscle. No statistically significant difference was found between the two groups. A planimetric evaluation of the nerve by axon circumference measurements, cross-sectional area of the axons, myelin area per axon and relative percentage of fibrous tissue was conducted. No differences were found between the two groups here either. These results indicate a similarity in functional nerve recovery after microsurgical repair using stitches or fibrin tissue adhesive.

Introduction

In clinical peripheral nerve microsurgery, acccurate adaptation and apositioning of the different fascicles is important. Epineural, perineural, and interfascicular techniques have been advocated. Microsurgical magnification and more precise knowledge of the intraneural anatomy have improved the results. Both clinical studies and animal models have failed to demonstrate a significant difference between epineural or perineural nerve repair [1], although perineural suturing gives better realignement of the fascicles and approximation of the perineurium. Animal studies in the rat have demonstrated that the number of reconnected axons does not differ after perineural or epineural nerve repair but the accuracy of reconnection is higher in perineural repair [2]. In perineural repair using stitches the following disadvantages could be observed compared with epineural repair:

1. More foreign body material is introduced when perineural stitches are used.
2. More intensive manipulation of the fascicles is required when perineural suturing is performed, compared with an epineural repair method, making the perineural repair more traumatizing.
3. Perineural suturing is a difficult and very demanding operation, requiring extensive skill.
4. Blood flow impairment at the suture line may be more pronounced when dissection and separation of the different fascicles is required for the perineural suturing technique.

Hypothetically, the use of fibrin glue could be advantageous regarding these points, but the fibrin glue anastomosis technique itself may have its own disadvantages [3] such as penetration of fibrin glue through the suture line and more pronounced connective tissue reaction induced by the glue, causing nerve compression.

A review of the literature on tissue glue showed a lack of physiological and histological evaluations of nerve and muscle function [4–7]. However, controversies still exist when comparing the results of these different techniques and, more importantly, in considering the effect of the placement of sutures inside the perineurium, possibly damaging the axon sprouting.

Also, suture placement may compress the blood supply to the different fascicles, thereby impairing the regeneration of the nerve ends after transection and repair. In clinical microsurgery, however, compromised vascularity, different degrees of crush injuries and different capabilities of nerve regeneration between various patients prevents a proper analysis of nerve function recovery. Therefore an experimental study was performed in the rat, comparing microsutures with tissue adhesive.

The aim of the experiment was to study the histology, physiology and electrophysiology of nerve repair, comparing nerve repair with perineural microsutures versus perineural tissue adhesive, and this in ideal experimental conditions for nerve repair. Such conditions should be: (a) no tension on the suture line; (b) no mismatches in reconnection or discrepancies between the fascicles; (c) an immediate repair after nerve section; (d) no blood between the nerve stumps.

Materials and Methods

In this experiment, 12 male Wistar rats, weighing 350–400 g, were used. Anesthesia was performed using intraperitoneal injection of pentutal.

The posterior tibial nerve was transected and repaired. On one side of the animal, the nerve repair was performed with microsutures (11-0 monofilament nylon). The other side was repaired with tissue adhesive (Tissucol). Using a Zeiss OPMI-6-D microscope, the posterior tibial nerve was approached. Only this fascicle was isolated from the sciatic nerve. Immediately after transection of the nerve, repair was undertaken. In the microsuture group three perineural individual stitches with 11-0 nylon at 120° were placed.

In the tissue adhesive group the nerve stumps from the freshly transected fascicle were brought together with two Dumont forceps, number 5 [3]. Care was taken that a maximum contact area between both nerve ends was obtained. Subsequently, a drop of the sealant solution and of the thrombin solution (250 IU/ml) were added. The sealant solution contains mainly fibrinogen, factor XII, fibronectin and albumin (45 mg clottable protein/ml) dissolved in an aprotinin solution (up to 150 KIU/ml). The thrombin solution consists of thrombin (250 IU/ml) dissolved in 20 mmol $CaCl_2$ solution. The importance of a high fibrinogen concentration and the addition of factor XII in regard to tensile strength of the fibrin glue has been stressed in previous work [3]. The conditions to obtain an optimal result using fibrin glue for nerve anastomosis were chosen based on previous studies [8]. We preferred a higher concentration of the antifibrinolytic agent aprotinin (150 KIU/ml instead of 50 KIU/ml) since very small amounts of fibrin glue were used and there was a fear of premature fibrinolysis. Stabilization of the nerve ends was maintained for 2 min. Fast reacting thrombin was added to the fibrinogen solution and a stable fibrin clot with chain cross-linking was formed within a few seconds.

Histological evaluation was performed 4 months postoperatively. Two biopsies were taken: one 3 mm proximal and the other one 3 mm distal to the suture line. On both histological sections the axonal diameter and the axonal area, correlated with the total area of the fascicle, were measured. Myelin sheet thickness was computed.

The first physiological evaluation was done 4 months postoperatively. The animals were anesthetized with Hypnorm (dog veterinary formula, Philips-Duphar B.V., Amsterdam, the Netherlands), 0.1 ml/100 g body weight intramuscularly. The gastrocnemius muscle was dissected and connected to a force transducer. The neurovascular pedicle was left intact during the whole procedure. The sciatic nerve was exposed over its five most proximal paravertebral millimeters. Here a bipolar stimulation electrode was placed under the nerve.

The contractile properties of the gastrocnemius muscle were measured with the muscle thermostatized at 37 °C in a paraffin mineral oil bath. After bringing the muscle under its rest tension, twitch tension (with a stimulus of 0.2 ms) and tetanic contractions at 10, 20, 35, 50, 80, 120, 150 and 200 Hz during 300 ms were evoked with stimuli which stimulated all the fibers in the nerve. All contraction curves were analyzed and stored in a computerized system; the analysis gave the maximum contraction force and maximum contraction velocity.

The maximum tetanic contraction force has the advantage over the twitch tension in that its size is less affected by facilitating (warming up effect) [9]. Between two stimulations the muscle can recover for at least 10 min in order to exclude fatigue as much as possible. The electrophysiological evaluation of the innervated muscle was performed by measuring the muscle evoked potentials. The registration was performed at the motor point of the muscle. Also the motor latency time was measured [10]. This parameter includes both the conduction time for the nerve and the muscle excitation time for the muscle excitation at the motor end plate. For physiological evaluation of the innervation, measurement of the tetanic maximum contraction capacity was performed and the maximum variation in force per time unit ($\Delta p/\Delta t$) is an approximation of the ideal physiological maximum contraction velocity (v 0) which should be measured without preload. The size of this value is related to the synchronization of the contraction of the different motor units. Physiological evaluation of the innervated muscle also was measured by measuring the maximum $\Delta p/\Delta t$ in a tetanic contraction. For statistical evaluation, an unpaired Student's *t* test was performed.

Results

Axonal Diameter

By comparing the axonal diameter an important decrease in axonal diameter was found between the proximal and the distal cross-section in both groups. In the suture group the axonal diameter measured 3 mm proximal to the anastomosis was 7.28 ± 1.75 μm and 4.33 ± 0.75 μm at 3 mm distal to the anastomosis side. For the tissue adhesive group the axonal diameter measured 3 mm proximal to the anastomosis was 6.71 ± 1.05 μm; 3 mm distal to the anastomosis the axonal diameter of the tissue adhesive group was 4.38 ± 1.04 μm.

Statistical analysis of axonal diameters proximal to the suture line revealed no statistically significant difference between both treatment groups ($p > 0.05$). The axonal diameter of the nerves 3 mm distal to the suture line did not show any significant statistical difference ($p > 0.05$) (Table 1).

Myelin Sheet Thickness

In the tissue adhesive group the myelin sheet thickness distal to the nerve repair was significantly thinner than in the suture group. Proximal to the anastomosis there was no significant difference in myelin sheet thickness between both groups. In the tissue adhesive group, the myelin sheet thickness was 0.85 μm proximal to the suture line and 0.92 μm distal to the suture line (Table 2). For the suture nerve repair group the myelin thickness was 1.88 μm proximal to the suture line and 0.22 μm distal to the suture line. The statistical difference between tissue adhesive and suture group was significant ($p < 0.05$).

Table 1. Axonal diameter

	Proximal		Distal	
Animal number	Fibrin glue	Micro sutures	Fibrin glue	Micro sutures
1	5,74	/	4,54	4,54
2	7,81	7,51	4,36	4,29
3	6,98	7,33	/	4,16
4	/	10,45	4,00	5,00
5	5,74	7,20	3,32	3,61
6	8,57	8,84	7,05	6,11
7	6,63	6,08	4,58	/
8	5,16	7,20	4,30	3,69
9	/	/	/	/
10	6,39	4,56	3,32	4,25
11	7,56	6,26	4,45	3,86
12	7,20	7,45	3,89	3,85
Mean	6,77	7,28	4,38	4,33
Standard deviation	1,05	1,57	1,04	0,75
	$p = 0.58$		$p = 0.51$	

Results are given in μm.

Table 2. Myelin sheath thickness

	Proximal		Distal	
Animal number	Fibrin glue	Micro sutures	Fibrin glue	Micro sutures
1	1,72	0,96	7,84	/
2	2,03	1,06	2,34	1,08
3	1,81	/	7,69	1,29
4	/	0,97	1,61	1,01
5	1,78	/	1,93	1,13
6	1,81	1,02	/	1,08
7	1,75	0,97	1,71	/
8	1,99	1,22	1,86	1,25
9	/	/	/	/
10	1,85	0,49	1,83	1,26
11	1,88	0,79	9,00	1,77
12	1,81	0,77	1,99	1,15
Mean	1,85	0,92	1,88	1,22
Standard deviation	0,11	0,21	0,91	0,22
	$p = 0.61$		$p = 0.008$	

Results are given in μm.

Table 3. Percent axonal area/total area

Animal number	Fibrin glue	Micro sutures	Fibrin glue	Micro sutures
1	48,68	/	48,68	44,54
2	73,82	64,31	37,25	45,61
3	61,24	68,12	/	48,74
4	/	108,23	17,39	56,24
5	56,21	67,13	27,90	33,95
6	58,98	63,53	64,46	46,96
7	70,47	71,36	37,78	/
8	53,90	65,33	39,25	38,43
9	/	/	/	/
10	65,22	48,85	36,59	39,88
11	65,13	65,11	46,01	44,57
12	63,74	70,34	40,31	35,03
Mean	61,73	69,26	39,36	43,39
Standard deviation	7,60	15,03	12,26	6,74
	$p = 0.51$		$p = 0.19$	

Axonal Area

Calculating the axonal area as a percentage of the total area, we found that proximal to the suture line there was no statistical significant difference between the tissue adhesive group and the suture group. In the tissue adhesive group 61.7 % ± 7.59 of the total area consisted of axons. In the suture group, 68.4 % ± 15.15 % of the total area consisted of axons (Table 3). Distal to the suture line, however, a much smaller axonal area was found: 9.15 % ± 2.02 % in the Tissucol group vs 10.94 % ± 1.53 % in the suture group.

Electrophysiological Evaluation

Electrophysiological evaluation of one nerve repaired with Tissucol gave the following results: The amplitude was 1582.4 g, the maximum $\Delta p/\Delta t$ was 42.37 g/ms. The latency time was 4 ms, the contraction time was 173 ms. The 50 % relaxation time was 123 ms and the area was 421457 g.

Regarding the electrophysiological evaluation of both repair groups, no statistical differences were found between both groups when the maximum tetanic contraction capacity was evaluated. In the suture group a maximum tetanic contraction of 1595 ± 324 g was measured (Table 4). In the Tissucol group a maximum tetanic contraction capacity of 1421 g ± 505 g was found. The p-value was < 0.005. However, the variations in the tissue adhesive group were higher and more extreme values were found in this group (2353 g and 571 g).

In studying the results of the maximum contraction velocity no statistical difference was found. The maximum contraction velocity indicates the number of motor units that are able to contract simultaneously. In the Tissucol group 42 ± 16 motor units were found vs 53 ± 19.48 in the suture group.

Table 4. Tetanic contraction

Animal number	Fibrin glue	Micro sutures
1	1223	1819
2	770	1012
3	571	1472
4	1471	1396
5	1582	1322
6	/	/
7	1311	2061
8	/	/
9	1837	1488
10	2353	1926
11	1556	1772
12	1537	1321
Mean	1421	1559
Standard deviation	505	324
	$p < 0.005$	

Results are given in grams.

Regarding the latency time we found an increase compared with the non-operated rats. This increase, however, was not statistically different from the nonoperated controls. However, this parameter does not tell us anything about conduction velocity since the muscle excitation time is included in this latency time. A latency time of 1.53 ms was found in the tissue adhesive group and 1.5 ms in the suture group.

Discussion

Either technique of microsurgical nerve repair, tissue adhesive or microsurgical sutures, provide only a 70% regeneration of nerve function. This despite optimal conditions of repair. In the rat no significant difference between microsutures and tissue adhesive was found in the contractile properties of the muscle. Also, histological evaluation of the nerve did not show any difference between the repair groups. A further detailed analysis of the electrophysiological properties of this type of nerve repair did not show any significant difference.

Only the thickness of the myelin sheet was significantly thicker in the suture nerve group. However, because we have not studied the conduction velocity of the nerves we cannot come to a final conclusion [11].

This experiment does not aim to prove whether one of the methods is superior, inferior, or equal. The use of fibrin glue for experimental nerve repair was first described by Young [12] and was used for the first time in the clinical situation by Kuderna in 1974 [in 8]. We wanted to document certain parameters of nerve regeneration in the rat model using the two different techniques. It was our opinion that the technique of gluing nerves was less traumatizing for the nerve and should give better results in nerve regeneration. There are two possible reason(s) why fibrin glue anastomosis failed: first, it could be that not the technique used for nerve repair but the intrinsic regenerative capacity of the nerve is the limiting factor in nerve regeneration [13]. Second, the quantities of fibrin glue used for nerve repair and its method of application are still far from ideal. We should be able to put a minimal amount of glue on exactly the right spot so that there is less glue used (less inflammatory reaction to the glue) and the glue that is used does not penetrate the nerve anastomosis.

In the clinical situation the use of fibrin glue has, besides the three advantages mentioned above, the additional advantage of being a fast and easy technique for nerve repair. With this study we think we can conclude that it is most unlikely that the results of nerve repair will differ on the basis of the technique used to repair the nerve. This result is in accordance with earlier clinical [14, 15] and experimental results [4, 5].

References

1. Orgel, MG (1987) Epineural versus perineural repair of peripheral nerves. In: JK Terzis (ed) Microreconstruction of nerve injuries. Saunders, Philadelphia, p 97
2. Brushart TM, Tarloui EC, Marsel MM (1983) Specificity of muscle reinnervation after epineural and individual fascicular suture of the rat sciatic nerve. J Hand Surg 8: 248–253
3. Matras H, Braun F, Lassmann H, Ammermeer HP, Mamoli B (1973) Plasma clot welding of nerves (experimental report). J Max Fac Surg 1: 236–247
4. Becker CM, Gueuning CO, Graff GL (1984) Sutures of fibrin glue for devided rat nerves: Schwann cell and muscle metabolism. J Reconstr Microsurg 1 (2): 139–145
5. Becker C, Gueuning CO, Graff G (1985) Réparation du nerf péripherique: intérêt des colles biologiques et de la suture épipérineurale dans les interventions tardives. Ann Chir Main 4 (3): 259–262
6. Boedts D (1982) Nerve anastomosis by a fibrinogen tissue adhesive. J Head Neck Pathol 3: 36–89
7. Cruz NI, Debs N, Fiol RE (1986) Evaluation of fibrin glue in rat sciatic nerve repairs. Plast Reconstr Surg 78 (3): 269–273
8. Matras H (1985) Fibrin seal: the state of the art. J Oral Maxillofac Surg 43: 605–611
9. Carlson FD, Walkie DR (1974) Mechanical aspects of muscular contraction. In: Carlson F, Walkie D (eds) Muscle physiology. Prentice-Hall, Engelwood Cliffs, p 33
10. Mackinon SE, Hudson AR, Hunter DA, Trued S (1986) Nerve regeneration in the rat model. Peripheral Nerve Repair Regeneration 1: 41–48
11. Schröder JM (1972) Altered ratio between axon diameter and myelin sheath thickness in regenerated nerve fibers. Brain Res 45: 49–65
12. Young JZ, Medawar DB (1940) Fibrin suture of peripheral nerves: measurement of the rate of regeneration. Lancet 239: 126–128
13. Lundborg G (1982): Regeneration of peripheral nerves: a biological and surgical problem. Scand J Plast Reconstr Surg Suppl 19: 38–44
14. Egloff DV, Narakas A (1983) Nerve anastomoses with human fibrin: preliminary clinical report (56 cases). Ann Chir Main 2 (2): 101–105
15. Bonnard C, Narakas A (1987) Comparison in clinical results of neurosynthesis when using microsutures of fibrin glue. Third Annual Meeting of the American Society for Reconstructive Microsurgery, San Antonio

Experimental Nerve Anastomoses with Fibrin Adhesive in a Rabbit Model

S. PALAZZI, J. VILA-TORRES, J. C. LORENZO, R. BORI, and E. RIU

Abstract

The aim of this study was to determine if the interposition of a 4 mm block of fibrin sealant in the nervus tibialis (internal popliteal nerve) of the rabbit would form a barrier which could stop or interfere with the passage of the axons.

A total of 24 adult rabbits nervi tibialis were placed in a microclamp, sectioned and separated by 4 mm. The gap between the two nerve ends was filled with fibrin sealant (Tissucol, Immuno). Some 8 weeks after the operation the rabbits were killed and their nervi tibialis removed. Histological studies and morphometric longitudinal and transverse studies showed that interposition of the block of fibrin sealant between the nerve ends did not act as a barrier or insurmountable obstacle of the passage of the axons. We conclude that fibrin sealant is a good experimental regeneration chamber because of the neurotization quota of 70%.

Introduction

Several experimental [1–4] and clinical [5, 6] studies have demonstrated the effective anastomosis of peripheral nerves by means of fibrin glue [7–10]. However, some nonetheless unsatisfactory results together with the hypothesis that fibrin adhesive placed between nerve fasciculi could create a closed barrier for axonal growth led us to perform the experiments described here. Our aim was to determine if the interposition of a 4 mm block of fibrin sealant (Tissucol, Immuno) between two ends of the nervus tibialis of the rabbit would form a barrier that could stop or interfere with the passage of the axons or their progression. The behavior and orientation of these axons when they cross the fibrin sealant block was also studied.

Material and Methods

A total of 24 adult New Zealand female rabbits, whose weight ranged between 1900 and 2100 g were used. Anesthesia was induced with ketamine (0.5 ml intramuscular injection in the forelimb) and continued by inhalation of sulfur

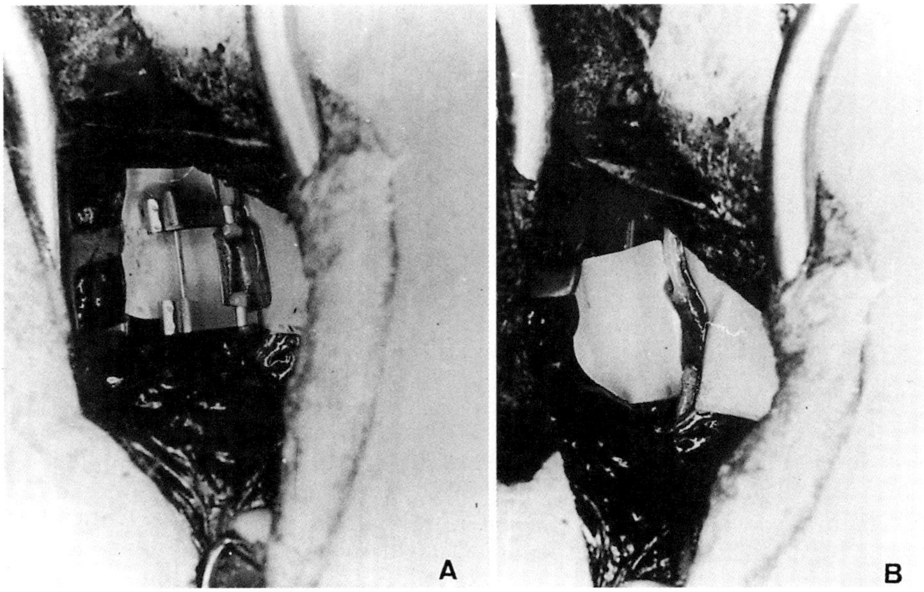

Fig. 1A, B. Nervus tibialis placed in the tube clamp **(A)**. Final aspect of the two nerve ends separated by Tissucol block **(B)**

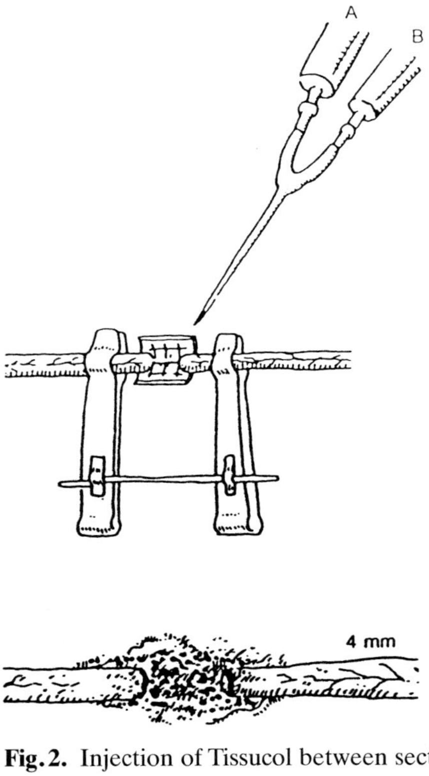

Fig. 2. Injection of Tissucol between sectioned nerve ends

ether (20 ml approximately) in a glass bell. After dissection, the nervus tibialis (internal popliteal nerve) was isolated and placed in a tube clamp (Fig. 1); neurotomy was then performed with microscissors. By means of retraction of the tube clamp branches, the nerve ends were separated by 4 mm. After that a two-component fibrin adhesive was placed between the ends with the aid of a double syringe (Fig. 2). Syringe A contained rabbit fibrinogen plus 0.5 ml aprotinin solution in a concentration of 100 KIU/ml. Syringe B contained 0.5 ml calcium chloride and thrombin 500 U/ml (catalyzed thrombin). The fibrin adhesive formed a "tube" conforming to the shape of the graduated silicon tube, which enclosed both nerve ends. The tube microclamp and the silicon tube were removed 3 min later and then the neurorrhaphy completed. The tensile strength of the anastomoses should be tested before skin closure by means of flexing and extending the limb. In ten rabbits, after nerve section an end-to-end anastomosis was performed to serve as controls. All rabbits received a single prophylactic dose of benzylpenicillin. The rabbits were killed 8 weeks later and a histological study of the removed samples was carried out. All nerve fragments were fixed on a 10% formalin-soaked tampon. Subsequently, the nerve fragments were sectioned longitudinally and soaked in paraffin. Afterwards, oriented histological sections from 3 to 5 μm, were obtained from each group. These were stained with hematoxylin-eosin and Masson's trichromic and Bodian's stain. Morphometric longitudinal and transverse studies were done using a Hewlett-Packard 1347 A Vectra ES/12 computer [11, 12]. Cell image analysis was performed by means of a Visilog 3.6.1 program (Computer Vision Software, Noesis, France).

Histological parameters (fibrosis, axons in the distal end) and the following morphometric characteristics were studied:

1. Analysis of axonal density
   a) Longitudinal sections
   b) Transverse sections
      - Total surface area of the section and the numerical axonal density (NAD) calculated as number of axons in a standard microscopic field divided by the displayed microscopic area
      - Peripheral (50% of external section)
      - Central (50% of the central section)
2. G index (ratio of axon size/fiber size)
3. Neurotization ratio (percent of axons in distal segment related to proximal, control segment)
4. Analysis of axonal shape
5. Analysis of axonal orientation and correlation between area, shape and orientation of axons in longitudinal sections

The values of the parameters were compared in the distal and proximal segments, the latter serving as the control. Stťdent's t test was applied to compare the two means. Pearsons's correlation test was used to assess the correlation of the data supplied by rose of directions.

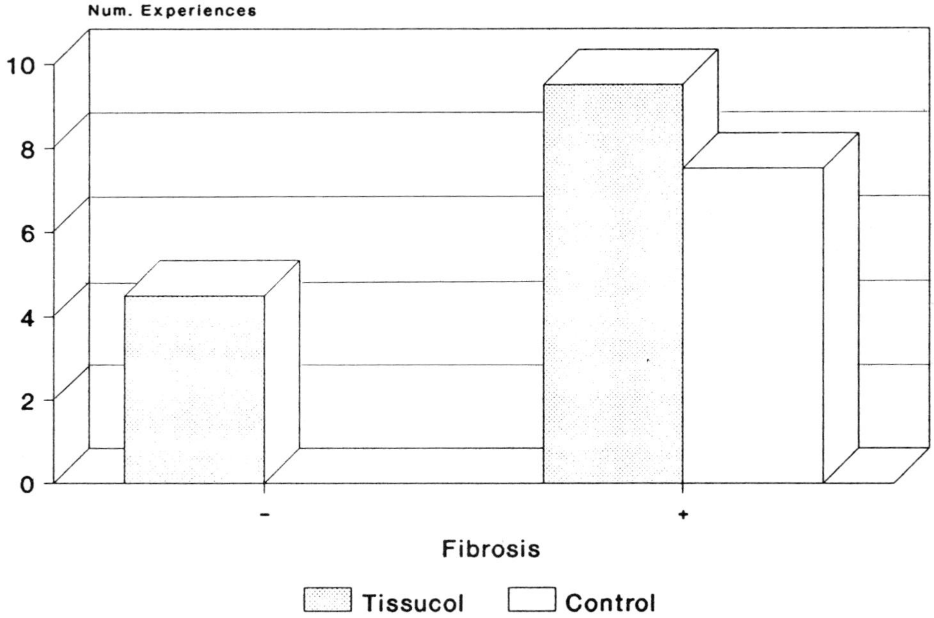

Fig. 3. Fibrosis in Tissucol and control groups in the sectioned nerve after 8 weeks

Results

In the histopathological study we observed a minor degree of fibrosis in the area (Fig. 3) and less foreign body reaction (Fig. 4) than in controls. Some 73 % of the samples showed axons in the distal end and 27 % presented tissue interposition; the orientation of these axons through the block of fibrin sealant was considered good in 87 % and fair in 13 %.

Regarding the morphometric evaluation performed in 16 specimens, the results were as follows (Table 1): Transverse analysis confirmed that 50 % of the axons were placed in the center of the section in the proximal and in the distal stump. There were no statistically – significant – differences NAD between the proximal and distal nerve stumps. A statistically highly significant correlation in NAD between ends was found, indicating that the higher the axonal density in the proximal stump, the higher the axonal density in the distal stump. Thus, fibrin sealant offers very little resistance to axon crossing. The G ratio was greater in the distal segment since the outer diameter of the fiber was smaller; the difference was statistically significant ($p < 0.02$). The explanation may be that the myelin sheath had not been totally restored at 8 weeks or that the restoration of normal structure in the distal segment was achieved earlier in the axons than in the myelin sheath.

In longitudinal sections, the analysis also did not find statistically significant differences in NAD between the proximal and distal nerve stumps. There were no statistically significant differences regarding recovery of normal axon

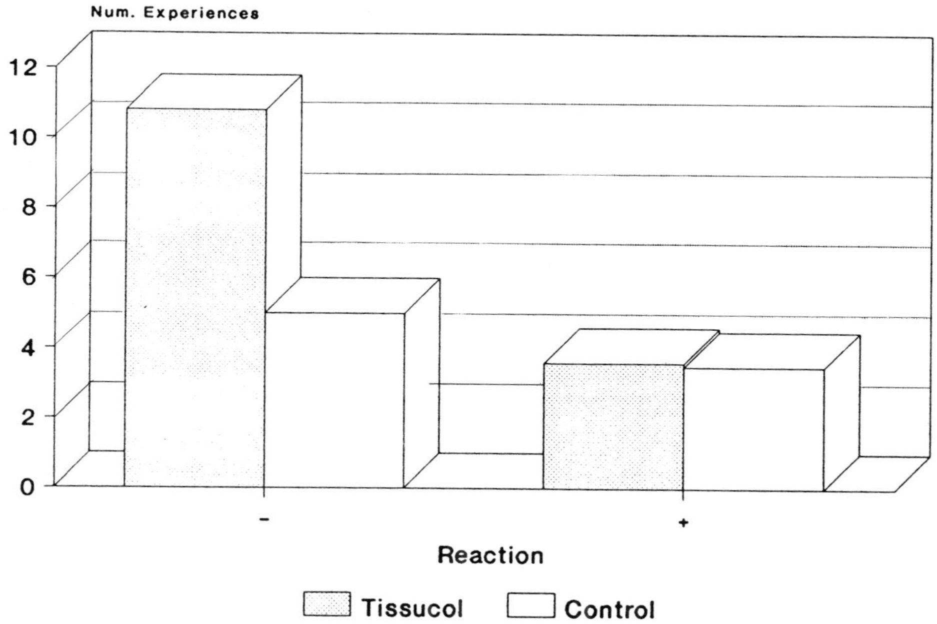

Fig. 4. Foreign body reaction in Tissucol and control groups in the sectioned nerve after 8 weeks

shape in the distal stump compared to the proximal one. A highly statistically significant correlation ($r = 0.97$, $p < 0.001$) was found regarding the spatial orientation of the axons between proximal and distal stumps. Through the fibrin sealant block the correlation was lower, probably indicating a slightly more disorganized architectural pattern (Fig. 5). There was a good correlation index among NAD, orientation and shape factors through the proximal, middle and distal segments. The neurotization ratio quantified in longitudinal and transverse sections, reached a level of around 70%. This indicates that 70% of the proximal axons reached the distal stump by crossing the fibrin sealant block, indicating little resistance.

Table 1. Summary of morphometric evaluations

Parameter	Statistical test	Significance
Axonal density in longitudinal sections	Student's t test	Not significant
Axonal density in transverse sections	Student's t test	Not significant
Shape factor	Student's t test	Not significant
Orientation	Pearson's test; $r = 0.97$	$p < 0.001$
G index	Student's t test	$p > 0.02$

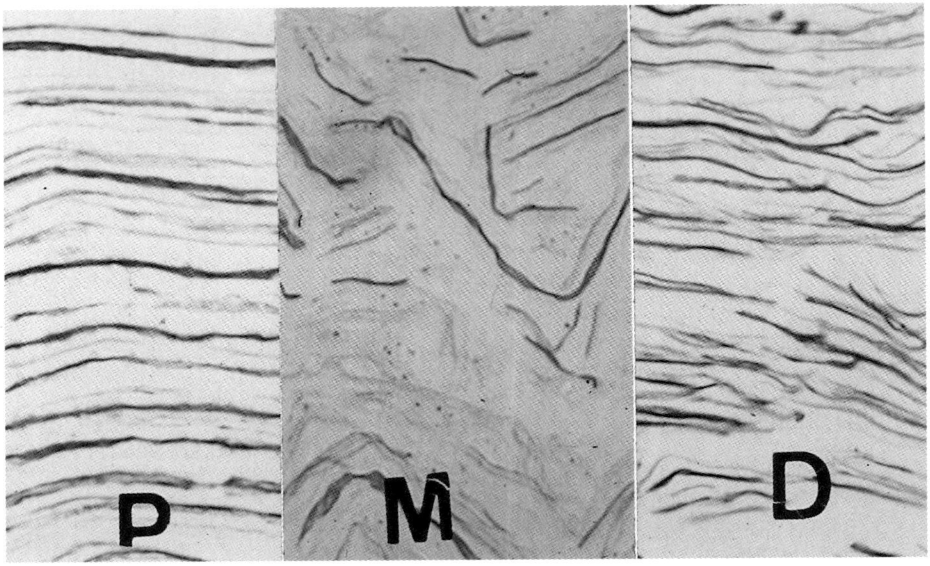

Fig. 5. After 8 weeks the nervus tibialis, separated by 4 mm of fibrin sealant, is removed. *P* proximal segment, axons are parallel. *M* medial segment corresponds to the passage of axons through the fibrin block; note the more disorganized architectural pattern. *D* Distal segment with restoration of the parallel pattern of the axons

Conclusions

Neurotomy and interposition of a 4 mm block of fibrin sealant produced dynamic structural changes. Morphologically, there was a minor degree of fibrin and less foreign body reaction than found in the control group.

Morphometric image analysis showed that axonal density, quantified in longitudinal and transverse sections, reached a neurotization quota of around 70%. The axonal density in the distal segment recovered its homogeneous spread. The G index indicated a higher index in the distal end of the nerve, due to the thinner myelin sheath. The shape of the axons was not affected by the fibrin block cross, and the longitudinal spatial orientation of the axons had fully recovered in the distal stump.

Thus, the interposition of a block of fibrin sealant between two nerve ends separated by 4 mm (three to four times the size of the nerve) is not a barrier or insurmountable obstacle to the passage of the axons. Fibrin sealant is therefore a good experimental regeneration chamber.

References

1. Young JZ, Medawar PB (1994) Fibrin suture of peripheral nerves. Lancet 239: 126–132
2. Matras H, Dinges HW, Mammoli B, Lassman H (1973) Non sutured nerve transplantation. J Max Fac Surg I: 37–40

3. Palazzi S, Borí R, Riu E, Lorenzo JC (1988) Anastomosis nerviosa experimental mediante el adhesivo de fibrina en el conejo. In: Doyma Sa (ed) XXX Ciclo de Sesiones Ortopédicas. Adhesivo de fibrina en Cirugía Orthopédica y Reconstructiva, pp 23–35
4. Smahel J, Meyer VE, Bachem U (1987) Glueing of peripheral nerves with fibrin: experimental studies. J Reconstr Microsurg 3: 211–220
5. Egloff DV, Narakas A (1983) Anastomoses nérveuses par fibrino-collage. Ann Chir Main 2: 101–115
6. Kuderna H (1979) Fibrin Kleber-System-Nervenklebung. Dtsch Z Zahn-Mund-Kiefer-Gesichts Chirug 3: 32s–35s
7. Duspiva W, Blümel G, Haas-Denk S, Wriedt-Lübbe I (1977) Eine neue Methode der Anastomosierung durchtrennter peripherer Nerven. Langenbecks Arch Chir [Suppl] 100
8. Palazzi S (1986) The use of fibrin sealant in nerve adhesions. In: Schlag G, Redl H (eds) Ophthalmology-neurology. Springer, Berlin Heidelberg New York, pp 186–191 (Fibrin sealant in operative medicine, vol 2)
9. Palazzi S, Palazzi C, Palazzi JL (1988) El empleo del adhesivo de fibrina en las anatómosis nerviosas. In: Doyma SA (ed) XXX Ciclo de Sesiones Ortopédicas. Adhesivo de Fibrina en Cirugía Ortopédica y Reconstructiva, pp 35–39
10. Tarlow IM, Denslow C, Swarz S, Pineles D (1943) Plasma clot suture of nerves. Arch Surg 47: 44
11. Jacobi P, Plos HG, Hams H, Haucke M, Aus HM (1987) Histometry of nerve fibers and nerve fiber autoradiography. In: Buerger G, Ploem JS, Goerttler K (eds) Clinical cytometry and histometry. London, pp 538–540
12. Russ JK (1990) Computer assisted microscopy. The measurement and analysis of images. Plenum, New York, pp 175–218

Outcome of Axonal Regeneration Following Rat Sciatic Nerve Transection Treated with End-to-End Microsuture or Fibrin Seal

B. Povlsen, P. Danielsson, and G. Nylander

Abstract

Fibrin is widely used to successfully secure nerve grafts in humans; however, it is seldom used in primary nerve repair, and the few reported animal studies show a high failure rate. These disappointing results prompted a prospective study to compare a new commercially available fibrin (Tisseel Duo 500 IU Thrombin) with a previously available product (Tisseel Kit 4 IU Thrombin). The two-stage study, using the rat sciatic nerve as a model, evaluated nerve end separation under an electron microscope in the three groups. In the first stage the two types of fibrin were compared. In the second stage, the sciatic nerves of those animals originally treated with Tisseel Duo were allowed to regenerate for a total of three months after which time they were sacrificed. After perfusion with glutaraldehyde, samples were taken from three branches of the sciatic nerve 30 mm distal to the original site of injury and examined under the electron microscope. Numbers of myelinated and unmyelinated nerve fibers were recorded in addition to measuring the diameter of the myelinated fibers. These results were then compared with controls of normal rats which had regenerated for three months after a controlled crash injury, and those which had the sciatic nerve sectioned and repaired using standard microsurgical techniques. There was no statistical difference in nerve regeneration between microsurgical repair and the use of Tisseel Duo fibrin in the primary repair of transsected peripheral nerves. All three types of nerve branch showed similar patterns of regeneration in the two types of repair. We conclude that neither Tisseel Duo, containing 500 IU thrombin, nor Tisseel Kit, containing 4 IU Thrombin, fail in the primary repair of transsected peripheral nerves in our model. This study also demonstrates equally good nerve repair and regeneration using Tisseel Duo and conventional microsurgical techniques.

Introduction

Nerve repair, nerve regeneration and functional recovery are of particular importance in hand surgery. In spite of seemingly adequate surgical treatment, cutaneous sensation of the hand, a function of fundamental importance, is usually not fully restituted after peripheral nerve transection [1, 2]. Often sensory function is not restituted beyond the level of "protective sensation" [3]. Hence, the study of structural and functional aspects of regeneration of sensory nerve fibers, at different levels is of considerable clinical interest [4, 5]. Most previous studies on this subject dealt with the sequence of events immediately above and below the site of injury [4].

Treatment of transected peripheral nerves and their poor outcome led Young and Medawar, in 1940 [6], to propose fibrinogen for nerve repair and the first use in humans was described in 1942 [7]. The fibrinogen, though, was not stable and further development was needed. A stable product was exhibited in 1972 by Millesi et al. and Matras et al. [8, 9], and the technique was then applied in humans on a greater scale by Kuderna-Matras in 1975 [10].

Since then, the technique has become regular practice in brachial plexus repair [11] and even in peripheral nerves with or without nerve grafting [10].

A major advantage has been the considerable time gain, stated by Narakas to be three-to-four fold [11]. Though several reports have been published casting doubt on the appropriate use in humans, Haase published, in 1986 [12], a rather negative result regarding the use of fibrin as a sole agent in nerve repair in rats. All distal anastomoses in nerve grafting had failed; the specifications of the fibrin were not mentioned.

The evaluation of functional outcome has mainly been at the muscular target organ [13, 14]. Very encouraging results have supported the fibrin glue technique, even when this technique has been used alone, in terms of regenerated muscular strength [11, 13, 15]. A more subjective assessment has supported the finding of sensory regeneration [11]. Very few animal studies have dealt with regeneration in sensory nerves, and the outcome of these has been contradictory [12, 16]. We have been unable to find previously described quantitative electron microscopy evaluations of axons following fibrin glue treatment of tributary nerve branches. The majority of studies have evaluated regeneration of muscular strength [15] and nerve conduction [13, 14] or used light microscopy to evaluate myelinated axons of the nerves [14, 16, 17].

In a previous study, we have used electron microscopy to analyze regeneration in sensory cutaneous and articular nerves and a motor branch [18]. We found significant differences in the regenerative pattern following transection and suturing.

The primary aim of this study was to examine the dehiscence rate in the sciatic nerve following neurotomy and treatment with fibrinogen, using either a new "ready-to-use" preparation (Tisseel Duo including 500 IE thrombin, Immuno AG, Austria) or a traditional "mixture" (Tisseel Kit including 4 IU thrombin). The second aim of this study was to examine the nerve branches and regeneration of their axon populations after neurotomy and treatment with one of the two fibrinogen preparations. The results will be compared to previously obtained results [18] in normal controls and following regeneration in response to a crush lesion to the sciatic nerve or neurotomy and subsequent treatment with microsuture. The branches examined were: the sural nerve (SN), supplying hairy skin on the hind foot; the lateral gastrocnemius nerve (LGN), supplying motor innervation to the lateral gastrocnemius muscle; and the posterior articular nerve (PAN), supplying the knee with sensory innervation. All are branches of the sciatic nerve [19, 20].

Material and Methods

Animals and Surgery

A total of 20, 3-month-old, female Sprague-Dawley rats were used. The rats were anesthetized with chloral hydrate (30 mg/100 g body weight i.p.) and the right sciatic nerve was exposed in the thigh. The nerve was cut about 5 mm below the site where it crosses the internal obturator muscle tendon. In ten rats the nerve was approximated with two pairs of microforceps and using a drop of Tisseel Duo over the transection site. In ten others, Tisseel-Kit was used. A single perineurial 10-0 nylon suture marked the anastomosis site. The wound was closed and the rats were allowed to move freely after surgery. Five rats from each of the two groups were examined 2 weeks postoperatively and dehiscence was noted. The five rats left were allowed to survive for 3 months.

Perfusion and Collection of Specimens

The animals were anesthetized with chloral hydrate, tracheostomized and ventilated with air. The heart was exposed and the animals were perfused with 500 ml Tyrode's solution, followed by 1000 ml 5% glutaraldehyde in a 300 mosm phosphate buffer containing 0.1 *M* sucrose. After perfusion, specimens were taken from the SN, the LGN and the PAN on the right side. The nerve specimens were postfixed overnight in glutaraldehyde, osmicated, dehydrated in acetone and embedded in Vestopal W [21].

Sectioning and Electron Microscopic Examination

Semi-thin and thin transverse sections were cut with a LKB Ultrotome IV, using glass or diamond knives. The sections were taken some 30 mm distal to the site of the lesion, this corresponding to the knee level. Semi-thin toluidine blue-stained transverse sections were used for orientation and general evaluation. Thin sections covering the entire cross-section of each nerve were collected on one-hole copper grids, coated with Formvar, contrasted with uranyl acetate and lead citrate, and examined in a JEOL JEM 1200 EX electron microscope. Montages of electron micrographs (x5000) were used for counting myelinated axons and for size measurements.

The numerical differences between regenerated and normal nerves indicated by the axon countings were statistically tested with the Wilcoxon test [22].

For each nerve and each experimental situation, measurements of myelinated fiber diameters (D, myelin sheaths included), and counts of obviously axon-related Schwann cell nuclei, were made on pictures form three cases.

Fiber diameters were calculated from cross-sectional areas determined with Videoplan 2 equipment [23].

Results

Two weeks postoperatively, five of the animals in each group were reexplored and the repair sites were exposed. All animals but one, in the Tisseel Kit group, had by 2 weeks a sciatic nerve in continuity and no neuroma.

It was therefore decided that rats from the Tisseel Duo group should proceed to electron microscopic evaluation.

Number of Myelinated Axons

Sural Nerve

In the fibrin sealed group (Fig. 1), the presence of small, irregularly shaped myelinated fibers is apparent. The number of Schwann cell nuclei per cross-section is 4.7-fold greater than the control level. Many Schwann cells exhibit empty troughs or lack an axonal relationship. Myelin degeneration products and macrophages are seen, and the amount of endoneural connective tissue seems to be increased. The number of myelinated axons is above normal (n = 1105, +30 %) (Table 1).

Nerve to the Lateral Gastrocnemius

Following sciatic neurotomy and fibrin seal the occurrence of small myelinated axons in the LGN is markedly increased and there are few large ones (Fig. 1). The myelinated axons tend to be irregularly shaped and may form minifascicles

Table 1. Numbers of myelinated axons in the sural nerve, the nerve to the lateral gastrocnemius muscle, and the posterior articular nerve of the knee joint

	Sural nerve	Nerve to the lateral gastrocnemius	Posterior articular nerve
Normal	841 (±117)	352 (±46)	86 (±6)
Crush	985 (±58)	498 (±47)	133 (±16)
Neur + Sut	1324 (±311)	513 (±122)	140 (±52)
Neur + fib	1105 (±94)	456 (±65)	141 (±49)

Normal, control animals; Crush, animals which have regenerated nerves during the 3 months following a crush lesion to the sciatic nerve; Neur + sut, following neurotomy and suture; Neur + fib, following neurotomy and fibrin seal.

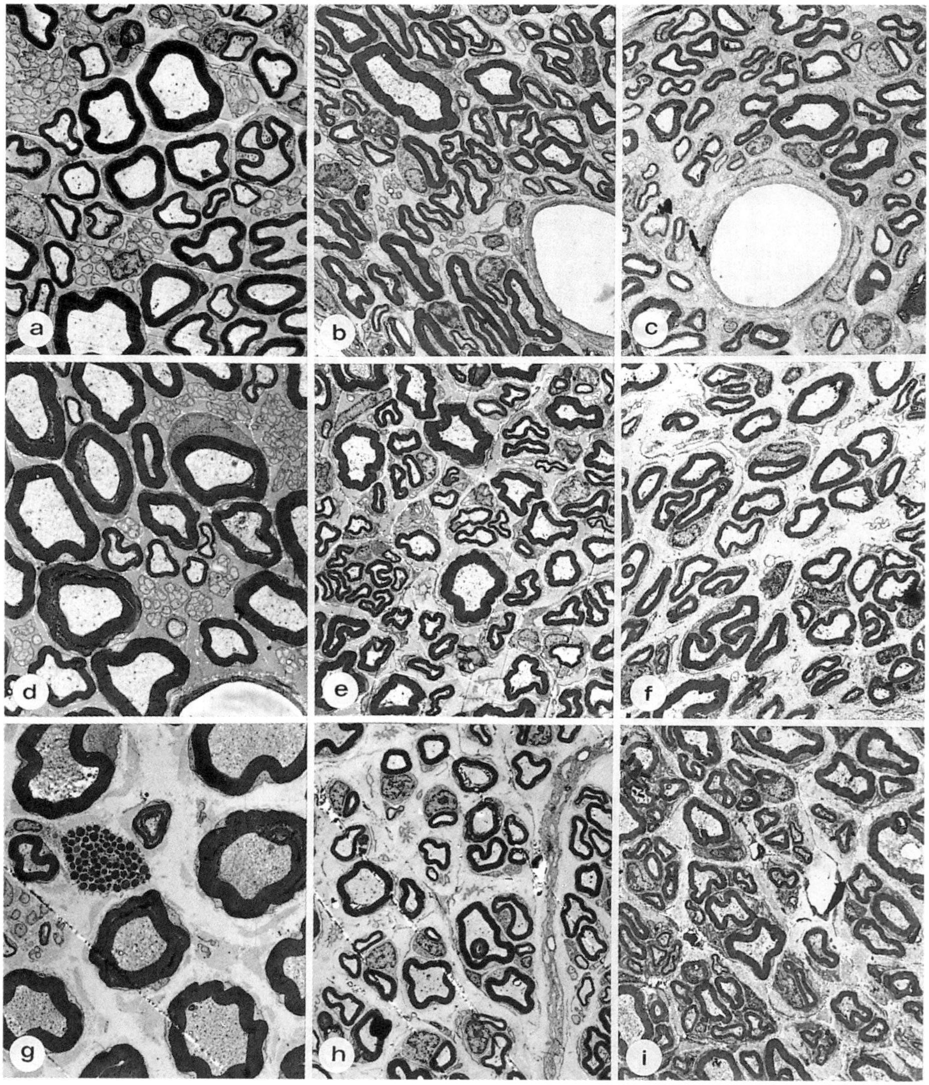

Fig. 1a–i. Electron micrographs showing representative fields from the cross-cut sural nerve **(a–c)**, nerve to the lateral gastrocnemius **(d–f)** and posterior articular nerve **(g–i)** in normal controls *(left row)*, 3 months following division and suture of the sciatic nerve *(middle row)* or approximated by fibrin seal *(right row)*. x5000

partly encircled by flattened cellular processes. The occurrence of Schwann cell nuclei per cross-section is 1.74-fold greater than the control level. Schwann cell profiles with empty troughs or devoid of an axonal association can be seen. The nerve exhibits some myelin remnants and macrophages, and there are more endoneural connective tissue components than normal. The average LGN exhibits 456 +30 % myelinated axons (Table 1).

Posterior Articular Nerve

In the fibrin sealed group, the presence of small, irregularly shaped, myelinated fibers is even more apparent (Fig. 1). The number of Schwann cell nuclei per cross-section is 1.66-fold greater than the control level. Some Schwann cells exhibit empty troughs or lack an axonal relationship. Myelin degeneration products and macrophages are found and the amount of endoneural connective tissue seems to be increased. In the average PAN the number of myelinated axons is clearly above normal (n = 141 +64 %) (Table 1).

Measurements

Sural Nerve

In the neurotomy and fibrin glue cases, the largest fibers reach 7.0 μm. Most myelinated axons are very small, with a peak at 2.0 μm. Some 73 % of them have diameters <3 μm.

Nerve to the Lateral Gastrocnemius

In the neurotomy and fibrin glue cases the largest fibers reach 7.0 μm. The myelinated axons are small with a peak at 2.0 μm. Some 73 % of them have diameters <3 μm.

Posterior Articular Nerve

In the neurotomy and fibrin glue cases the largest fibers reach 5.0 μm with a peak at 2.0 μm. Most of the myelinated axons are very small. Some 90 % of them have diameters <3 μm.

Discussion

The first part of this study examined dehiscence following neurotomy in rats treated with either Tisseel Duo or Tisseel-Kit. The outcome was determined following apposition of the nerve ends with a drop of either of the two and allowing the animals unrestricted movement until examination 2 weeks post operatively. In the Tisseel-Kit group the failure rate was one of five (in addition to one of five from the animals that did not proceed to electron microscopic investigation) and none in the Tisseel-Duo group (five at 2 weeks and five at 12 weeks). These findings may explain why the previous results by Haase [12], exhibited such a high failure rate, all distal anastomoses in nerve grafting having failed; however, the exact type of Tisseel was not mentioned. In fact, none of the proximal anastomoses failed in the study by Haase; but the closer the anastomoses were located to the knee joint, the higher was the failure rate. It is also possible that Tisseel Kit was used, which may have a shorter tensile strength, predicting a higher failure rate [6, 8, 9]. It therefore seems that Tisseel Duo does not exhibit a significant failure rate, even when the transected nerves are not immobilized, contrary to common practice for most peripheral surgery in humans. It is therefore interesting to investigate the outcome in tributary nerves of the sciatic nerve following treatment with Tisseel Duo. Many authors have questioned the fibrinogenic effect of Tisseel in nerve repair and this subject has been investigated by several groups [13, 17]. However, the negative impact of increased fibrin interaxonally is still unclear.

We have previously analyzed the electron microscopy images of regeneration in sensory cutaneus and articular nerves and in a motor branch [18] following crush or transection and suture of the sciatic nerve. We found significant differences in the regenerative pattern. This report examines axonal regeneration in three sciatic nerve branches following neurotomy and fibrin sealing (Tisseel Duo). The SN, LGN and PAN are all branches of the sciatic nerve [18].

Previous results [18] showed that the normal SN contains an average number of 29 axon-related Schwann cell nuclei per cross-cut SN. Control specimens contain an average of 841 myelinated axons (Table 1). Following regeneration after a sciatic crush lesion the number of myelinated axons is higher than normal ($n = 973$, +16 %) (Table 1). In the sutured group, the amount of endoneural connective tissue seems to be increased and for the average SN the number of myelinated axons is clearly above normal ($n = 1324$, +41 %) (Table 1). The increase in myelinated axons following suture of the SN has also been noted by others [24, 25]. Measurements show that the myelinated fibers in the neurotomy/suture cases reach 6.5 μm for the largest fibers, but most myelinated axons are very small. Some 73 % of them have diameters <3 μm.

In the normal LGN, numerous large myelinated axons dominate. Scattered small myelinated axons and tiny clusters of unmyelinated axons also occur. There are, on the average, 14 axon-related Schwann cell nuclei per cross-cut nerve and 352 myelinated axons (Table 1). In crushed cases there are 499 myelinated fibers; the absolute numbers are 42 % higher than in controls (Table 1). Following sciatic neurotomy/suture the average LGN exhibits 514 myelinated axons. The absolute numbers are abnormally high (45 %) (Table 1). In controls the LGN exhibits a bimodal myelinated fiber size distribution. In divided/sutured cases the size distribution is unimodal; there is a peak at about 2 μm, and the maximum diameter, which few fibers reach, is 6–7 μm. Some 70 % of all myelinated axons have diameters <3 μm.

The normal PAN is composed of 86 myelinated axons (Table 1). In crushed cases the myelinated axons have increased by 56 % ($n = 134$). Following neurotomy and suture the myelinated PAN have 140 myelinated axons, the number of myelinated axons is +62 % (Table 1). Myelinated fibers in the normal PAN exhibit a size range of 1–8 μm, and a distinct peak at 3 μm. Some 40 % of all myelinated fibers are <3 μm in diameter. Nerves from crushed cases show similar size ranges, but the spectra are shifted to the left, and 72 % of all myelinated axons are <3μm. A similar picture is at hand following neurotomy and suture.

With respect to the fibrin glue situation, our results show that the SN deviates from normal similar to a neurotomy/suture lesion, both more than following a crush lesion. Though the number and diameter of the SN axons following fibrin sealing show a regenerative tendency, resembling after a crush injury, the situation is nonetheless significantly different. Also, in the LGN the myelinated axons increase in the fibrin glue situation, but to a lesser extent than seen after suture, though not significantly different. The PAN exhibits a marked numerical increase in myelinated axons (+63 %). In terms of numbers of Schwann cell nuclei per cross-section, degeneration products, occurrence of endoneural collagen and fibroblasts, no significant differences were seen compared to conventional suture.

Our study results regarding SN following crush injury or neurectomy and suture confirm previous observations [24, 25] and support our results regarding neurectomy and fibrin glue in the SN, the LGN and the PAN.

Turning now to the effects of sciatic nerve injury on fiber sizes, our measurements show that the LGN is clearly smaller after neurotomy, but the technique of rejoining does not result in any significant difference; nevertheless, fewer very small myelinated fibers are found in the sealed group. Previous results from crush injury of the SN and the LGN show that there are large fibers, although the range is normal. Following neurotomy, of the SN the range is reduced and the spectrum is markedly shifted towards smaller sizes, but no significant difference is found between suturing and sealing. In the PAN the range is clearly reduced after either neurotomy/suture or fibrin glue.

We would have expected to find more axons with maximum or higher diameters in the fibrin seal treated group, especially in the LGN, based on previously described higher conduction velocities following fibrin sealing [13]. It is possible however, that the regeneration pattern in our study differs from that of the facial nerve of the cat [13], which may carry motor branches among the larger diameter axons.

Conclusion

Our observations confirm that primary peripheral nerve repair with fibrin seal (Tisseel Duo) does not exhibit an increased anastomosis failure rate compared to neurotomy and suture. The quantitative regenerative pattern of myelinated axons in branches to different target areas appears not to change when the neurotomy is approximated by fibrin glue rather than by microsuture.

Tisseel Duo seems promising, but further functional analysis of sensory regeneration is desirable, before it can be advocated in humans.

References

1. Önne L (1962) Recovery of sensation and pseudomotor activity in the hand after nerve suture. Acta Chir Scand Suppl 300: 1–69
2. Sunderland S (1978) Nerves and nerve injuries. 2nd edn. Churchill Livingstone, Edinburgh

3. Dellon AL (1981) Evaluation of sensation and reeducation of sensation in the hand. Williams and Wilkins, Baltimore
4. Lundborg G (1988) Nerve injury and repair. Churchill Livingstone, Edinburgh
5. Mumenthaler M, Schliack H (1991) Peripheral nerve lesions. Diagnosis and therapy. Thieme, Stuttgart
6. Young IZ, Medawar PB (1940) Fibrin suture of peripheral nerves. Lancet 239: 126
7. Seddon HJ, Medawar PB (1942) Fibrin suture of human peripheral nerves. Lancet 2: 87
8. Matras H et al. (1972) Zur nahtlosen interfaszikulären Nerventransplantation im Tierexperiment. Med Wochenschr 122: 517
9. Millesi et al. (1972) Experimentelle Untersuchungen zur Heilung durchtrennter peripherer Nerven. Chir Plast 1: 174
10. Kuderna H, Matras H (1975) Die klinische Anwendung der Klebung von Nervenanastomosen bei der Rekonstruktion verletzter peripherer Nerven. Wien Klin Wochenschr 87: 495
11. Narakas A (1988) The use of fibrin glue in repair of peripheral nerves. Orthop Clin North 19: 187–199
12. Haase J et al. (1986) Use of fibrin seal (Tisseel/Tissucol) in peripheral nerve surgery: an experimental rat model. In: Schlag G, Redl H (eds) Ophthalmology-neurology. Springer, Berlin Heidelberg New York, pp 196–197 (Fibrin sealant in operative medicine vol 2)
13. Bento RF, Miniti A (1989) Comparison between fibrin tissue adhesive, epineural suture and natural union in intratemporal facial nerve of cats. Acta Otolaryngol Suppl (Stockh) 465: 4–35
14. Herter T (1988) Problems of fibrin adhesion of the nerves. Neurosurg Rev 11: 249–258
15. Nishihira S, McCaffrey TV (1989) Repair of motor nerve defects: comparison of suture and fibrin adhesive techniques. J Otolaryngol Head Neck Surg 100: 17
16. Crutz NI et al. (1986) Evaluation of fibrin glue in rat sciatic nerve repairs. J Plast Reconstr Surg 78 (3): 369–373
17. Smahel J, Meyer VE, Bachem U (1987) Gluing of peripheral nerves with fibrin: experimental studies. J Reconstr Microsurg 3 (3): 211–218
18. Hildebrand C, Povlsen B (1991) Cutaneous, muscular and articular nerve fibre regeneration after rat sciatic nerve lesions. Soc Neurosci Abstr 378: 17
19. Greene EC (1963) Anatomy of the rat. Hafner, New York
20. Hebel R, Stromberg MW (1986) Anatomy and embryology of the laboratory rat. BioMed, Wörthsee
21. Berthold CH (1968) A study on the fixation of large mature feline myelinated ventral lumbar spinal root fibres. Acta Soc Med Ups 73: 1–36
22. Petrie A (1987) Lecture notes on medical statistics, 2nd edn. Blackwell, London
23. Karnes J, Robb R, O'Brien PC, Lambert EH, Dyck PJ (1977) Computerized image recognition for morphometry of nerve attributes of shape of sampled transverse sections of myelinated fibers which best estimates their average diameter. J Neurol Sci 34: 43–51
24. Jenq C-B, Coggeshall RE (1984) Regeneration of axons in tributary nerves. Brain Res 310: 107–121
25. Jenq C-B, Coggeshall RE (1985) Numbers of regenerating axons in parent and tributary peripheral nerves in the rat. Brain Res 326: 27–40

Fibrin Glueing of Peripheral Nerves

J. SMAHEL and V. E. MEYER

Abstract

Experiments were carried out on rats to compare fibrin glueing of nerves with suturing. For this purpose, the sciatic nerves were transected and the cut ends were joined either by glueing with Tissucol or with an epineurial suture. The slower acting type of Tissucol fibrin glue was used with 100 units of aprotinin. A piece of silicone tubing cut in half lengthwise provided a useful splint for the glueing procedure; it stabilized the nerve stumps and prevented adhesion to surrounding structures. Separation of the stumps did not occur in any of the glued nerves. Histologic studies performed up to 6 months after the operation showed no appreciable difference in either healing or the outcome of nerve regeneration between glued and sutured nerves. The equivalence of the two methods was substantiated by the absence of statistically significant differences on electrophysiologic determination of the latency period and amplitude of compound action potentials. Fibrin glueing did not give superior results regarding nerve regeneration but the method is attractive for clinical purposes since it is simpler and less time-consuming than suturing.

Introduction

Reuniting severed nerves by using fibrin glue instead of traumatizing sutures dates back to the experimental work of Young and Medawar [1] and Tarlov et al. [2] in the early 1940s. However, the method remained purely experimental until the 1970s, when Matras et al. [3, 4] and Kuderna [5] developed it further. An essential factor in this development was the introduction of a simplified sealing system, Tissucol by (Immuno AG, Vienna). Experimental [6–9] and clinical [10, 11] studies on this subject have been published recently. The introduction of a simplified sealing system led us to review the method with respect to joining severed nerves and compare results with those achieved by suturing [12].

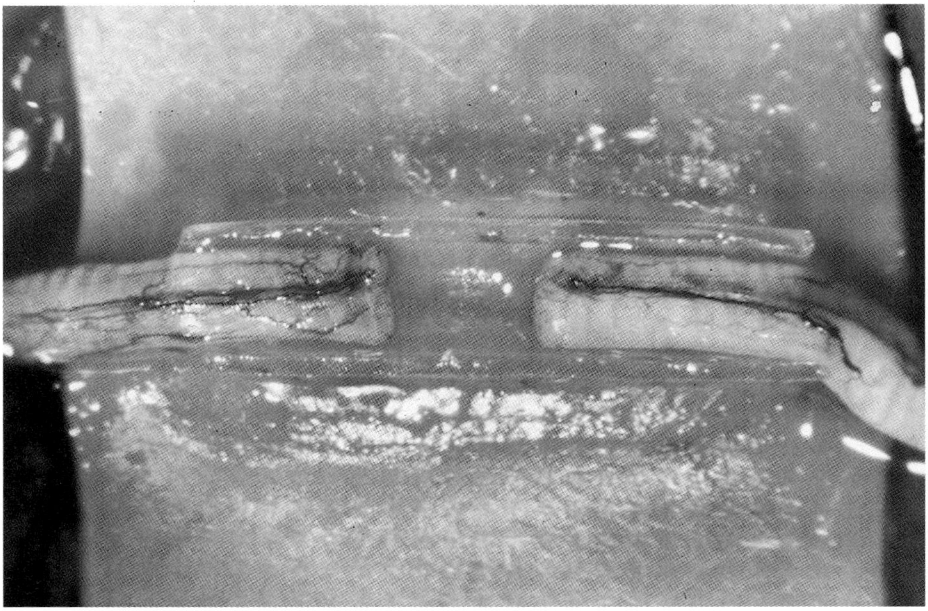

Fig. 1. Device for glueing of divided nerves

Material and Methods

A total of 48 female rats, weighing between 250 and 280 g, were used for the comparative study. Under general anesthesia, the sciatic nerve was transected bilaterally. On one side, alternating between left and right, the cut ends were joined by sutures consisting of four epineurial stitches using 10-0 nylon. On the other side, the transected nerves were glued with Tissucol. The slower acting type (L) of Tissucol was used, with 100 units/ml of aprotinin. The glueing procedure was facilitated by a simple device consisting of fine silicone tubing cut in half lengthwise and attached to a rubber base (Fig. 1). The device was removed after waiting for 5 min to allow for fibrinogen polymerization. To protect the joining against any forceful pull, a relief suture was made with 8-0 nylon thread, anchoring it very superficially in the epineurium.

Electrophysiologic and histologic assessment was made 1 and 3 days, 1, 2, 3, and 4 weeks, and 3 and 6 months after the operation. Six nerve pairs were available for comparison on each occasion. Electrophysiologic assessment consisted of determination of the latency and amplitude of the compound action potentials of the repaired nerves. For this purpose, the repaired nerves were exposed and 25 mm segments excised. The distance between the bipolar stimulating and recording electrodes was 18 mm, with the junction site at the center. A stimulus of 10 mA/0.05 ms was applied. When these measurements had been taken, the nerve segments were reduced to 15 mm in length, fixed in formalin, and embedded in paraffin by the usual method. The serial longitudinal sections were stained with hematoxylin and eosin and by the Hansen modification of van Gieson's method. Holmes' modification of Bodian's method was used for silver impregnation.

Results

Histologic examinations of glued and sutured nerves in the first week after the operation revealed the characteristic features of the two techniques. Glueing does not assist coaptation of the stumps but merely fixes their position achieved by approximation. As the cut surfaces of peripheral nerves are apt to be convex, contact may be inadequate at the periphery (Fig. 2). If the nerve is sutured, the thread can be pulled tight to achieve close contact in the periphery. However, this inevitably means compression of the central part of the nerve and potential twisting of the nerve fibers.

Histologic studies showed no appreciable difference in healing or outcome of nerve regeneration between glued and sutured nerves. Both groups characteristically showed some degree of variation in the histology, but this reflected differences in the execution of the method rather than in the method itself.

On the first day after surgery, the distribution of the fibrin coagulum was still clearly recognizable in the glued nerves. By the third day relatively little remained of the fibrin, and proliferation of neurofibroblasts and Schwann cells into the gap was noted in both groups. At this point, the axons in the proximal stump had thickened, whereas the distal stump showed the usual axon and myelin sheath degeneration. One week after surgery, no fibrin was noted

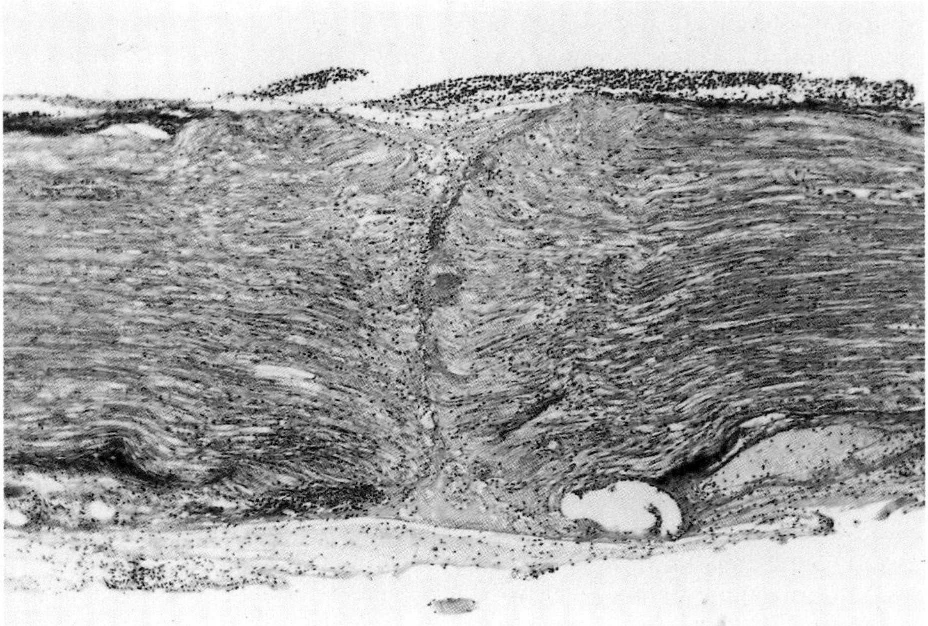

Fig. 2. Glued nerve stumps, 1 day after surgery. van Gieson, x65

around the glued nerves. The connection between the stumps had been reestablished in both groups and the proliferating axons were beginning to penetrate into the distal stump. In the following weeks the number of bridging axons increased steadily, with the axons extending further into the distal stump. Three weeks after the operation they had penetrated about 10 mm in both groups. Three months after the operation, healing of the juncture was essentially complete (Fig. 3). The juncture had been bridged by numerous axons which largely ran parallel in the glued nerves. Axons were less uniformly arranged in sutured nerves, as sutures presented an obstacle that axons had to overcome. The number of axons appeared to be about the same for both groups.

The equivalence of the two methods of nerve repair was substantiated by the absence of statistically significant differences on electrophysiologic examination. Determination of latency periods, reflecting the mean rate of conduction for all regenerated axons, showed that, after 6 months, conduction of the impulse in the repaired nerves was almost the same as for nerves that had not been operated on; this applied to both groups. Determination of the amplitude of compound action potentials, indicating the number of regenerated axons showed amplitudes well below the mean for nerves that had not been operated on. The differences between glued and sutured nerves were not significant.

Discussion

Peripheral nerve repair with the fibrin glue Tissucol was found to be technically simple, requiring considerably less time than suturing. The slower-acting thrombin solution (L) was used in preparing the fibrin glue, adding 100 units/ml of aprotinin. At this aprotinin concentration, degradation of the fibrin glue takes 5–7 days, which is just the time required to establish the connective tissue link between the stumps. Earlier reports showed the aprotinin concentration to be a crucial factor in nerve repair [5].

A piece of silicone tubing cut in half lengthwise provided a useful splint for the glueing operation: it stabilizes the nerve stumps and prevents adhesion to surrounding structures. Postoperative immobilization was not feasible and we therefore applied a relief suture. No special studies were done to establish the need for this measure. However, none of the glued nerves separated again. The use of a relief suture provided useful addition information. Examinations done at the conclusion of the healing period showed that the suture was not in tension, indicating that the glued nerve had not stretched in the healing process (Fig. 3).

According to our study, there is no appreciable difference between the two methods of nerve repair, regarding the healing process and the end effect. This agrees with the observations in other studies performed under comparable experimental conditions [6–9].

Fibrin glueing did not give superior results regarding nerve regeneration, but the method seems attractive for clinical purposes, its execution being simpler and less time-consuming than that of the suturing technique. The method

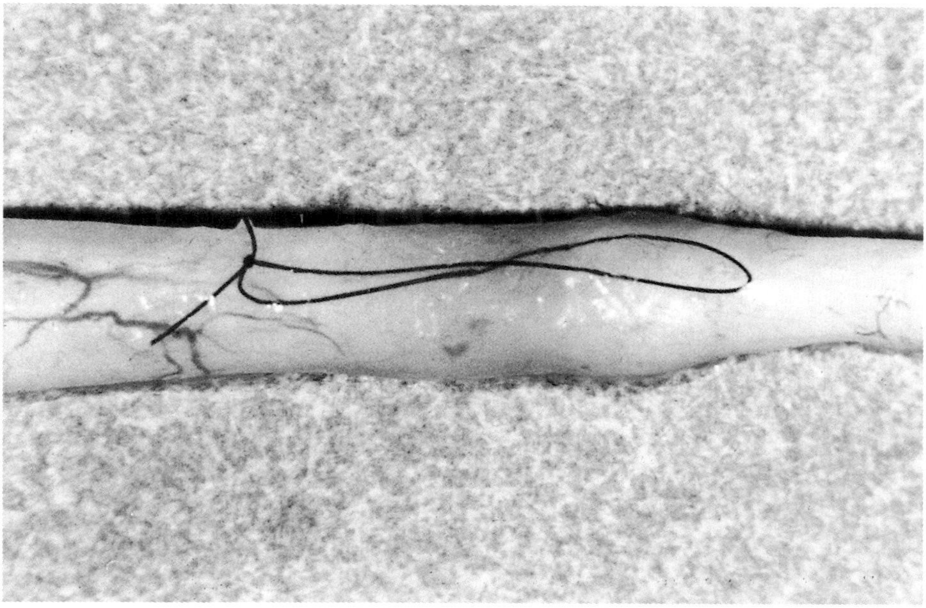

Fig. 3. Complete healing of a glued nerve 3 months after surgery. The relief suture in situ is shown

of glueing may lead to a considerable shortening of the operating time, especially in brachial plexus surgery where we use it more or less in the same way as advocated by Narakas [11].

References

1. Young JZ, Medawar PB (1940) Fibrin suture of peripheral nerves. Lancet 239: 126–128
2. Tarlov IM, Denslow C, Swarz S, Pineles D (1943) Plasma clot suture of nerves. Arch Surg 47: 44–58
3. Matras H, Dinges HP, Lassmann H, Mamoli B (1972) Zur nahtlosen interfaszikulären Nerventransplantation im Tierexperiment. Wien Med Wochenschr 122: 517–523
4. Matras H, Braun F, Lassmann H, Ammerer HP, Mamoli B (1973) Plasma clot welding of nerves (experimental report). J Max Fac Surg 1: 236–247
5. Kuderna H (1979) Nervenklebung. Dtsch Z Mund Kiefer Gesichts Chir 3: 32–35
6. Becker CM, Gueuning CO, Graff GL (1984) Sutures of fibrin glue for divided rat nerves. J Reconstr Microsurg 1: 139–145
7. Benfrech E, Alnot JY, Henin D (1989) Etude expérimentale des sutures et greffes nerveuses de nerf sciatique chez le rat par fibrino-collage. Ann Chir Main 8: 296–299
8. Boedts D (1982) Nerve anastomosis by a fibrinogen tissue adhesive. J Head Neck Pathol 3: 86–89
9. Moy OJ, Peimer CA, Koniuch MP, Howard C, Zielezny M, Katikaneni PR (1988) Fibrin seal adhesive versus nonabsorbable microsuture in peripheral nerve repair. J Hand Surg 13A: 273–278
10. Egloff DV, Narakas A (1983) Anastomoses nerveuses par fibrino-collage. Ann Chir Main 2: 101–115

11. Narakas A (1988) The use of fibrin glue in repair of peripheral nerves. Orthop Clin North Am 19: 187–199
12. Smahel J, Meyer VE, Bachem U (1987) Glueing of peripheral nerves with fibrin: experimental studies. J Reconstr Microsurg 3: 211-218

A Combination of Fibrin Sealant and Nerve Growth Factor Accelerates the Regeneration of Leading Sensory Fibers in Experimental Peripheral Nerve Repair

A. Worseg, L. Zeng, G. Leichtfried, H. Redl, and G. Schlag

Abstract

The purpose of this study was to investigate whether (1) fibrin sealant (FS) can be combined with nerve growth factor (NGF) in order to release NGF from the biodegradable fibrin matrix to the surrounding area; (2) the presence of NGF locally could affect axonal outgrowth in the early phase of regeneration.

A total of 36 (three groups of 12) male Sprague-Dawley rats, each weighing 300–320 g, were used. Sciatic nerves were transected at the level of the great trochanter and coapted with two standard epineural sutures. FS matrix with (FS-NGF group) and without (FS group) NGF (2 μg/ml) was placed around the suture line and the surrounding area. Suture only served as a control group. Regeneration was measured by pinch test at 3, 4 and 6 days after surgery. In addition, the NGF release characteristics from the NGF-FS matrix were investigated in vitro by ELISA. The results revealed significantly faster regeneration of the leading sensory nerves at 3 and 4 days postoperatively in both the FS and FS-NGF groups than in the suture group only. In vitro, a high peak of NGF release was seen within the first 18 h; afterwards release remained slow for 2 weeks. We conclude that: (1) FS as a carrier can be combined with exogenous NGF without destroying the activities of the NGF; (2) local application of a FS-NGF matrix could be beneficial for regeneration of leading sensory fibers in peripheral nerves.

Introduction

The regenerative capacity of transected peripheral nerve is influenced by many factors, such as good mechanical coaption by careful microsurgical technique, regenerative potential of the proximal nerve, and neurotrophic messages from the distal nerve stump. Nerve growth factor (NGF), which has been isolated from mouse sarcomas, is an important physiological regulator of neurons of the peripheral nervous system [1]. Sensory and sympathetic neurons derive NGF trophic support from the target organs which they innervate [2]. In addition to these targets of innervation, another important source of NGF for the peripheral nervous system is the nerve itself. Schwann cells of peripheral nerves contain NGF immunoreactivity and are induced to produce NGF by macrophage-derived interleukin-1 following axotomy [3]. Another important property of NGF is its ability to direct growing or regenerating axons of sensory and sympathetic fibers along its concentration gradient (neurotropism) [4].

It is well known that the fibrin sealant (FS) matrix can act as a carrier for antibiotic agents, forming an absorbable matrix for local use in chronic infections. The purpose of this study was to combine FS matrix with exogenous NGF to create a local environment of NGF with its neurotropic and neurotrophic properties. A rat sciatic nerve model was used to check whether the presence of FS and NGF may be beneficial to axon outgrowth. In addition, the in vitro release characteristics of exogenous NGF in the FS matrix were analyzed.

Materials and Methods

Animal Model

A total of 36 male Sprague-Dawley rats (three groups of 12), each weighing 300–320 g, were used. Anesthesia was carried out by intramuscular administration of ketamine – Rompun combination. The sciatic nerve was sharply transected at the level of the great trochanter and then coapted with two standard epineural sutures (10-0 nylon). A FS matrix, consisting of 0.1 ml sealant protein (mainly fibrinogen) and 0.05 ml of a 500 IU/ml thrombin solution in $CaCl_2$ (4 mmol/l) enriched with 0.05 ml NGF (8 μg/ml saline solution), was placed in the interstice between the sutures and surrounding area (NGF-FS group). FS matrix alone served as the second group (FS group). Epineural suture only served as the control group (SUT group).

Axonal regeneration was measured by pinch test at 3, 4 and 6 days after surgery.

Pinch Reflex Test

The pinch test reliably demonstrates the extent to which most rapidly growing sensory axons (pain fibers) have regenerated [5, 6].

Rats were anesthetized superficially and the sciatic nerve was exposed from the hip distally to well beyond the division of the tibial and peroneal branches. Using microtip forceps the nerve was firmly pinched, beginning at the distal end and then approaching the junction site until a reflex response was obtained. The first reflex is usually a contraction of the flexors of the same side (withdrawal reflex). The pinch reflex point, which represents the position of the distal end of the fastest growing axons, was marked with a nylon cerclage suture and the nerve was removed together with adherent tissue and immediately placed on millimeter graph paper. The distance between suture site and pinch reflex point was measured and recorded.

Nerve Growth Factor Release In Vitro

A series of 0.4 ml FS-NGF (2.5 μg/ml) matrix samples were incubated at 37 °C for 42 h with 2 ml phosphate buffer with or without 7.5 μg/ml urokinase. Samples were taken at 0, 18, 30 and 42 h and centrifuged; the supernatant was stored at –30 °C for ELISA determination.

ELISA for Nerve Growth Factor

The microtitration plate wells were coated with mouse-derived monoclonal anti-NGF antibodies in 100 μl of 0.1 *M* sodium bicarbonate buffer (pH 9.2) for 24 h at 37 °C. The residual free binding sites were then blocked with 250 ml of phosphate-buffered saline solution (PBS containing 1 % bovine serum albumin) for 1 h at 37 °C and incubated with 100 μl of NGF sample and standard in PBS (containing 1 % bovine serum albumin) for 2 h at 37 °C. This was followed by incubation with rabbit-derived polyclonal anti-NGF antibodies in 100 μl of PBS for 2 h at 37 °C and with peroxidase-conjugated antibodies to rabbit immunoglobulins in 100 μl of PBS for 1 h at 37 °C. Fresh immunoperoxidase substrate solution, 0.4 mg/ml ortho-phenylenediamine in 0.1 *M* sodium citrate buffer, pH 5.0, containing 0.02 % H_2O_2 was prepared and 100 μl was added per well, developed for 15–20 min in the dark and discontinued with 10 μl of 25 % H_2SO_4. We measured the optical density with an ELISA reader at 450 nm and washed each step properly.

Results

At 3 and 4 days postoperatively regeneration of the leading sensory axons (pain fibers) in the rat sciatic nerve, as measured by pinch reflex test, showed significant ($p < 0.05$) improvement in the NGF-FS and in the FS group compared to the SUT group.

At 6 days postoperatively there was faster regeneration of the leading axons in the NGF-FS group than in the FS and SUT groups; however, the difference was not statistically significant (Table 1).

Table 1. Regeneration of the rat sciatic nerve by pinch testing

	Regeneration distance (mm)		
	3 days	4 days	6 days
Suture	6.1 ± 0.3	7.8 ± 0.3	10.6 ± 0.3
Suture + FS	7.7 ± 0.4*	9.0 ± 0.4*	10.6 ± 0.3
Suture + FS + NGF	7.8 ± 0.3*	9.6 ± 0.3*	11.4 ± 0.6

FS, fibrin sealant; NGF, nerve growth factor.
Values are mean ± SE; $n = 12$. * $p < 0.05$.

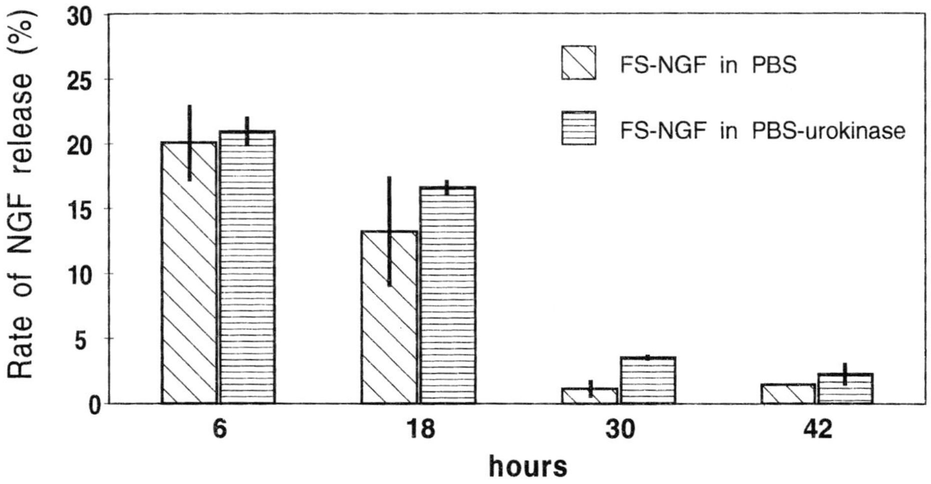

Fig. 1. ELISA determination for nerve growth factor *(NGF)* release in vitro: 33.3 %–37.6 % of total amount of the NGF added in the fibrin sealant *(FS)* was released within the first 18 h. No significant differences were found in a high or low fibrinolytic milieu

In vitro the release of NGF from FS matrix showed a high peak within the first 18 h. Afterwards only slow release was detected till the FS clots were dissolved totally in about 2 weeks (Fig. 1). No differences were found whether the FS matrix was in a high or low fibrinolytic milieu.

Discussion

In the present study a FS matrix enriched with exogenous NGF was used to accelerate axonal outgrowth after nerve transection and primary suture in a rat sciatic nerve model.

FS is widely used in peripheral nerve repair for its adhesive properties. A common procedure is the combination of FS with microsutures to provide good nerve contact. Long-term results indicate a similarity in functional nerve recovery after microsurgical repair using stitches or fibrin tissue adhesive alone [7]. It has been previously demonstrated that FS is not a barrier for the passage of axons [8, 9]; therefore, FS which gets between the nerve stumps application onto the anastomosis, will not disturb axonal regeneration.

In this study a FS matrix, with its biodegradable properties, was evaluated as a carrier for exogenous NGF as a method to release active factors to the local surroundings. Detection and quantification of the actual release of NGF in vivo represents a methodological problem; therefore, the release characteristics of NGF in the FS matrix were determined in vitro (Fig. 1). The data clearly indicate a microenvironment of high concentrations of exogenous NGF during the first days following local application of the FS-NGF matrix in vivo.

The time course after permanent nerve transection suggested a biphasic pattern of neurite-promoting activity. The activity decreased to a minimum by 14 days after transection and then increased again to a new maximum at 51 days [10].

High concentrations of exogenous NGF may compensate for the initial decrease of autogenous neuronal growth factors.

The significantly increased regeneration rate of the fastest sensory fibers was only obtained during the first and fourth day after transection. An explanation may be the half life of the fibrin sealant in rat soft tissue, which was demonstrated to be 2.82 +/- 0.31 days [11]. About 50 % of the added FS matrix is lysed and absorbed in the first 3 days, probably leading to a weakening of the temporary support framework for the growth cones [12].

Summary

Fibrin sealant matrix as a carrier can be combined with exogenous NGF to form a biodegradable matrix without destroying neurotopic and neurotrophic activities. The matrix releases active factors locally and creates a neurotropic and neurotrophic microenviroment in the early phase of nerve regeneration. Local application of a combination of FS and NGF accelerates sprouting of the leading sensory fibers in the early phase.

References

1. Levi-Montalcini R (1987) The nerve growth factor 35 years later. Science 237: 1154–1162
2. Korsching S, Thoenen H (1983) Nerve Growth Factor in sympathetic ganglia and corresponding target organs in the rat: correlation with density of innervation. Proc Natl Acad Sci USA 80: 3513–3516
3. Heumann R et al. (1984) Differential regulation of mRNA encoding Nerve Growth Factor and its receptor in rat sciatic nerve during development, degeneration and regeneration: role of macrophages. Proc Natl Acad Sci USA 84: 8735–8739
4. Polizis MJ, Ederle K, Spencer PS (1983) Tropism in nerve regeneration in vivo: attraction of regenerating axons by diffusible factors derived from cells in distal nerve stumps of transected peripheral nerves. Brain Res 261: 109–117
5. Young JZ, Medawar PB (1940) Fibrin suture of peripheral nerves: measurement of the rate of regeneration. Lancet 2: 126–128
6. Arntz C, Kanje M, Lundborg G (1989) Regeneration of the rat sciatic nerve after different conditioning lesions: effects of the conditioning interval. Microsurgery 10: 118–121
7. Boeckx W, Stockmanns F, Guelinckx P (1992) Microsurgical and physiological evaluation of nerve repair with microsuturing versus tissue adhesive: presented on update and future trends in fibrin sealing in surgical and non surgical fields, 15–18 Nov 1992, Vienna
8. Pallazi S (1986) The use of fibrin sealant in nerve adhesions. In: Schlag G, Redl H (eds) Ophthalmology-neurosurgery. Springer, Berlin Heidelberg New York, pp 186–191 (Fibrin sealant in operative medicine, vol 2)
9. Zeng L, Leichtfred G, Dinges HP, Schlag G, Redl H (1994) An experimental study of peripherial nerve repair with a biodegradable neurotropic and neurotrophic matrix. Eur J Plast Surg 17: 228–232

10. Windebank AJ, Poduslo JF (1986) Neuronal growth factors produced by adult peripheral nerve after injury. Brain Res 13: 199–212
11. Millesi H (1990) Review article: peripheral nerve surgery today: turning point or continuous development? J Hand Surg [Br] 15: 281–287
12. Pflüger H (1986) Principles of fibrin sealant. In: Schlag G, Redl H (eds) Ophthalmology – neurosurgery. Springer, Berlin Heidelberg New York (Fibrin sealant in operative medicine, vol 2), pp 39–50
13. Weiss P (1941) Nerve patterns: the mechanics of nerve growth. Growth, Third Growth Symposium 5: 163–203

Experimental Peripheral Nerve Repair with Nerve Growth Factor and Fibrin Sealant Matrix: Functional and Morphological Evaluation

L. Zeng, W. Öhlinger, H. Redl, and G. Schlag

Abstract

In this study, a fibrin sealant (FS) matrix, with or without nerve growth factor (NGF), has been used to improve the recovery of severed peripheral nerves. A total of 30 male Sprague Dawley rats, weighing 250–270 g each, were used. Sciatic nerves were transected at the level of the great trochanter and then connected with two standard epineurial sutures. FS with NGF (2 μg/ml) was placed in between the nerve anastomosis and the surrounding area (group NGF-FS). The second group was treated with FS only (group FS). The control group had only sutures (group SUT) ($n = 10$/group). Functional recovery process (up to 12 weeks) was evaluated by serial walking-track analysis and calculation of the rate of muscle atrophy (RMA). Morphological evaluation was analyzed by immunohistochemical staining with an antibody to neurofilament (APAAP method). The behavioral data, expressed by the sciatic function index (SFI) and the toe spreading index (TSI), indicated significant improvement in the group NGF-FS at the ninth week postoperatively ($p < 0.05$). The RMA was significantly lower ($p < 0.05$) in the group NGF-FS at the 12th week. Histologically, a better regeneration ($p < 0.05$) of neurites was found in group FS. We concluded that local application of a combination of FS and exogenous NGF may be useful for neuritic regeneration and subsequent functional recovery.

Introduction

It has been demonstrated that nerve growth factor (NGF) is an essential protein for growth and maintenance of peripheral sympathetic and sensory neurons [1, 2]. During early periods of ontogenesis, it has been also reported that peripheral motor neurons might be sensitive to NGF [3, 4]. For example, the sciatic nerve, which contains axons from motor, sympathetic and sensory neurons, is known to be one of the pathways of NGF transport. Injury to the rat sciatic nerve leads to a dramatic increase in local NGF synthesis and NGF mRNA expression [5, 6] and to accumulation of NGF distal to the injury [7].

It has also been previously demonstrated that a fibrin sealant (FS) matrix can be a source of some antibiotics against chronic infections. Local application of this combination of fibrin matrix and antibiotics leads to the formation of microenvironment with a gradient of antibiotic concentrations [8]. Our previous in vitro study has revealed that FS can also be combined with exogenous NGF, which can be released from the mixed matrix to surrounding areas without loss of the NGF activities for up to 14 days [9]. It has been further demonstrated in an in vivo study that local application of a FS matrix enriched with NGF may accelerate regeneration of the leading sensory fibers in the early phase (up to 4 days after nerve transection) in the rat sciatic model, as evaluated by the pinch reflex test [10].

The purpose of the present study was to check whether the presence of NGF-FS may improve functional recovery and morphological regeneration following sciatic nerve transection over 3 months.

Materials and Methods

Animal Model

A total of 30 male Sprague-Dawley rats, each weighing 250–270 g, were anesthetized by intramuscular administration of a Ketamine-xylazine combination (Ketalar-Rompun) (Ketalar, 50 mg/kg body weight; Rompun 16 mg/kg body weight). With an aseptic technique, one side of the sciatic nerve trunk was exposed through a 2 cm longitudinal incision. The nerve was sharply transected at the level of the greater trochanter, then repaired with two standard epineurial sutures (10-0 nylon). The FS matrix, which consisted of 0.1 ml sealant protein solution (mainly fibrinogen) and 0.05 ml of a 500 IU/ml thrombin solution in $CaCl_2$ (40 mmol/l) with 0.05 ml NGF (8 μg/ml saline), was placed in between the nerve anastomosis and the surrounding area (group NGF-FS). The FS matrix without NGF served as the second group (group FS). The sutures only served as a control (group SUT) (n = 10/group). The nonoperated contralateral leg of each animal was used as the control in the walking-track analysis. After the operation the animals were kept separately in single cages without immobilization and with free access to water and food.

Functional Evaluation

Walking-track analysis [11, 12] was assessed serially by footprint records and described by the sciatic function index (SFI) and the toe spreading index (TSI). The hindlimb footprint of each animal was obtained by wetting the feet with film developer and allowing the animal to walk along a path of X-ray film exposed to ambient light. The test was performed every 3 weeks for a 12 week period. From the footprints manual measurements were blindly made of the print length (PL), the intermediary toe abduction (IT; second to fourth toe), and the toe spread (TS) (first to fifth toe) of the normal (N) and experimental (E) sides (NPL, NIT, NTS, EPL, EIT, ETS) (Fig. 1). The SFI and TSI were calculated by using the following formulas:

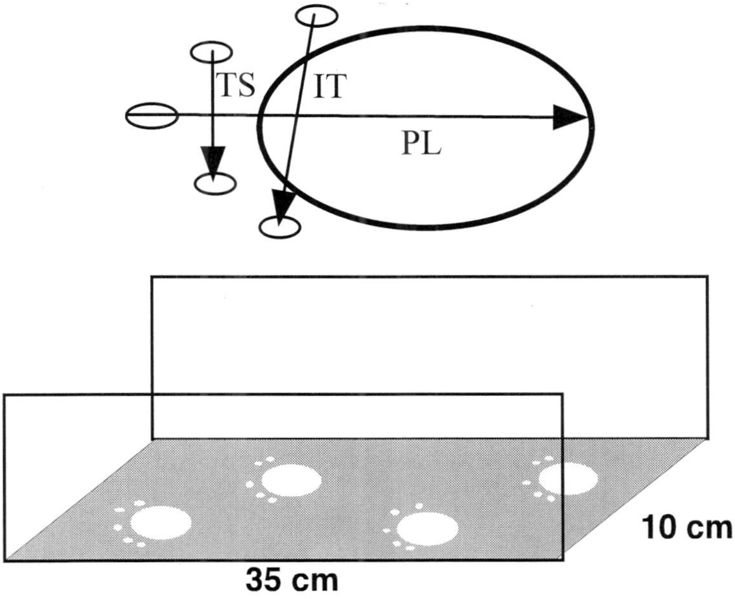

Fig. 1. The walking-track analysis

$$SFI = -38.3 \left(\frac{EPL\text{-}NPL}{NPL}\right) + 109.5\left(\frac{ETS\text{-}NTS}{NTS}\right) + 13.3\left(\frac{EIT\text{-}NIT}{NIT}\right) - 8.8$$

$$TSI = (NTS\text{-}ETS)/NTS$$

Index "0" indicates normal function for both the SFI and TSI. An index of "1" for TSI and "–100" for SFI signify total impairment.

Ratio of muscle atrophy (RMA) was calculated from the tibialis anterior (TA) muscles, which are innervated by the sciatic nerves, on both the normal (N) and experimental (E) side. The muscles were isolated and harvested at their origins and weighed to the nearest 0.01 g. The ratio was calculated according to the following formula: RMA = (NTA-ETA)/ETA.

Morphological Sampling and Evaluation

After walking-track analysis, deep anesthesia was established by intramuscular injection of Ketalar-Rompun. A perfusion system was set up by separately inserting a catheter into the right jugular vein for inlet of the perfusion and left external carotid artery for outlet of the perfusion. Gravity perfusion was performed with 100 ml 10 % 0.1 *M* phosphate-buffered formalin solution (pH 7.4) with a flow speed of 5 ml/min. After perfusion, the nerve segments were carefully removed and placed in the same solution overnight and embedded in paraffin. After predigestion of paraffin sections with pronase, longitudinal sections (5 µm thick) were stained with a monoclonal antibody against neurofilament (mouse-anti-human neurofilament, DAKO 1:50, cross-reacting with rat nerve fibers) using the alkaline phosphatase anti-alkaline phosphatase (APAAP) method. Sections were examined in a double-blind fashion. Semi-quantitative analysis, according to the orientation and regeneration of the fibers at the transected sites, were assessed.

Statistics

All measurements were carried out in a double-blind fashion, and codes were broken only after analysis of the data had been performed. The values (scores) from morphological evaluation were tested for significance by Fisher's exact test. The data (means ± SEM) from functional evaluations were submitted to an analysis of variance followed by a *t* test for group comparisons. The calculations were performed using SAS Software Release 6.03 (SAS, Cary, NC). Differences in the experimental means were considered to be significant if $p < 0.05$.

Results

Regarding the functional evaluation, both the SFI and the TSI showed some improvement in both the NGF-FS and FS groups at 6 weeks compared to the SUT group. However, significant improvement of both indices was obtained in the NGF-FS group only at 9 weeks after the operation (Figs. 2, 3).

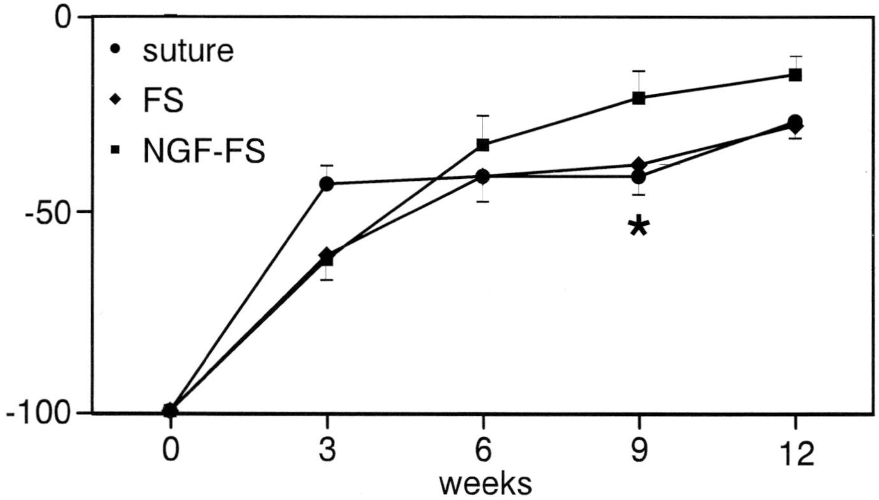

Fig. 2. Sciatic function index (SFI) calculated by walking track analysis. Values are means +/– SEM; $n = 10$. *Zero* reflects formal function; *–100* represents no function. *FS*, fibrin sealant; *NGF*, nerve growth factor

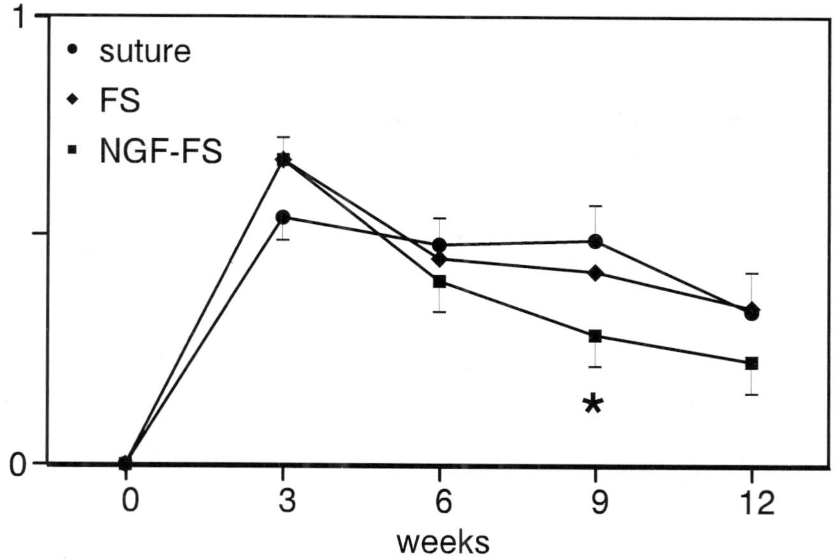

Fig. 3. Toe spreading index (TSI) evaluated by walking track analysis. Values are means +/– SEM; $n = 10$. *Zero* reflects formal function; *1* represents no function. *FS*, fibrin sealant; *NGF*, nerve growth factor

The RMA was significantly lower in the NGF-FS group ($p < 0.05$) than in the group SUT at 12 weeks after surgery (Fig. 4).

Morphologically, there was good and excellent regeneration and orientation of regenerated fibers at the transected sites encountered in both NGF-FS

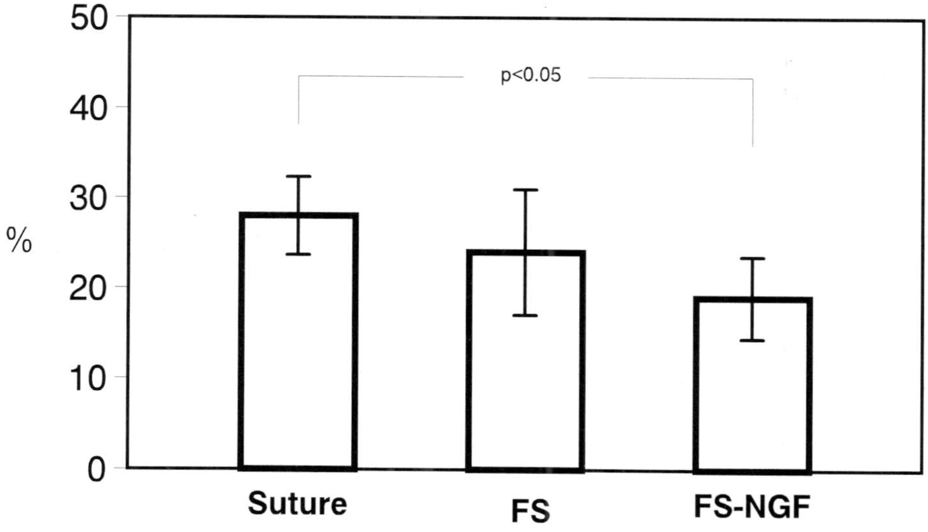

Fig. 4. Ratio of corresponding muscle atrophy (tibialis anterior) at 12 weeks after surgery; $n = 10$

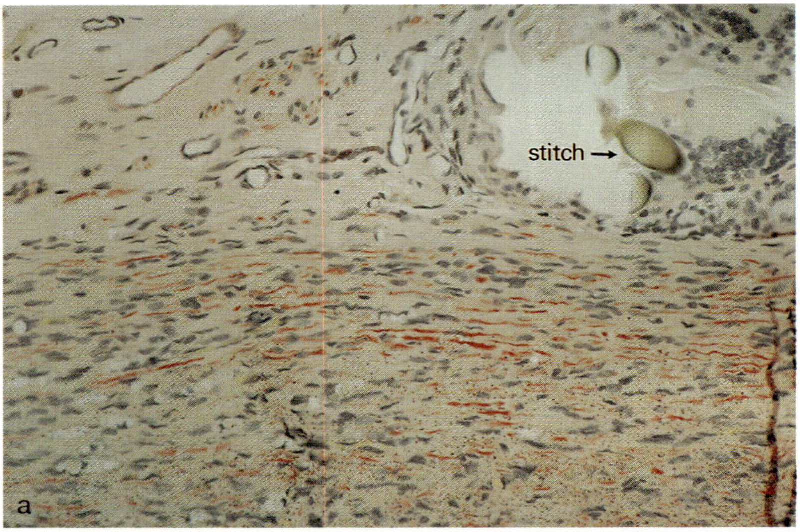

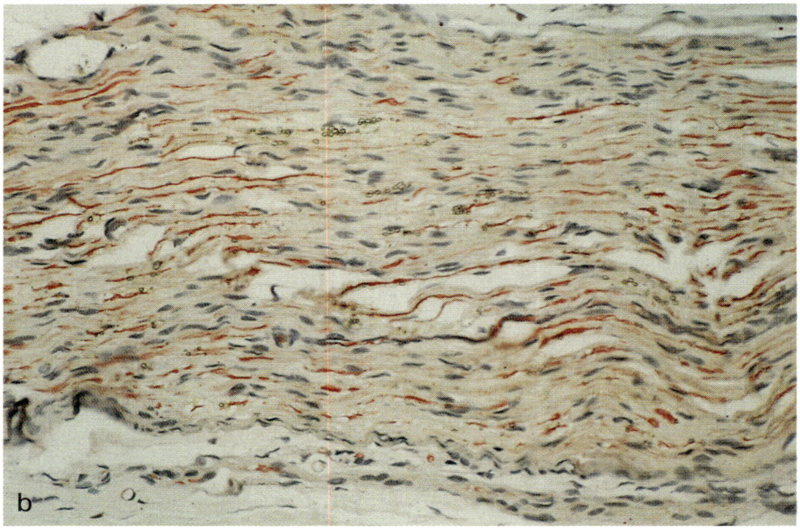

Fig. 5 a–d. Longitudinal sections of the rat sciatic nerve which were transected and repaired. **a** Good orientation and regeneration of the axons at the transected site in group FS; **b, c** good orientation and regeneration of fibers in the group nerve growth factor-fibrin sealant *(NGF-FS)*, immunostaining with **(b)** and without **(c)** counterstain; **d** poor orientation and regeneration in the group SUT. Neurofilament staining; × 20

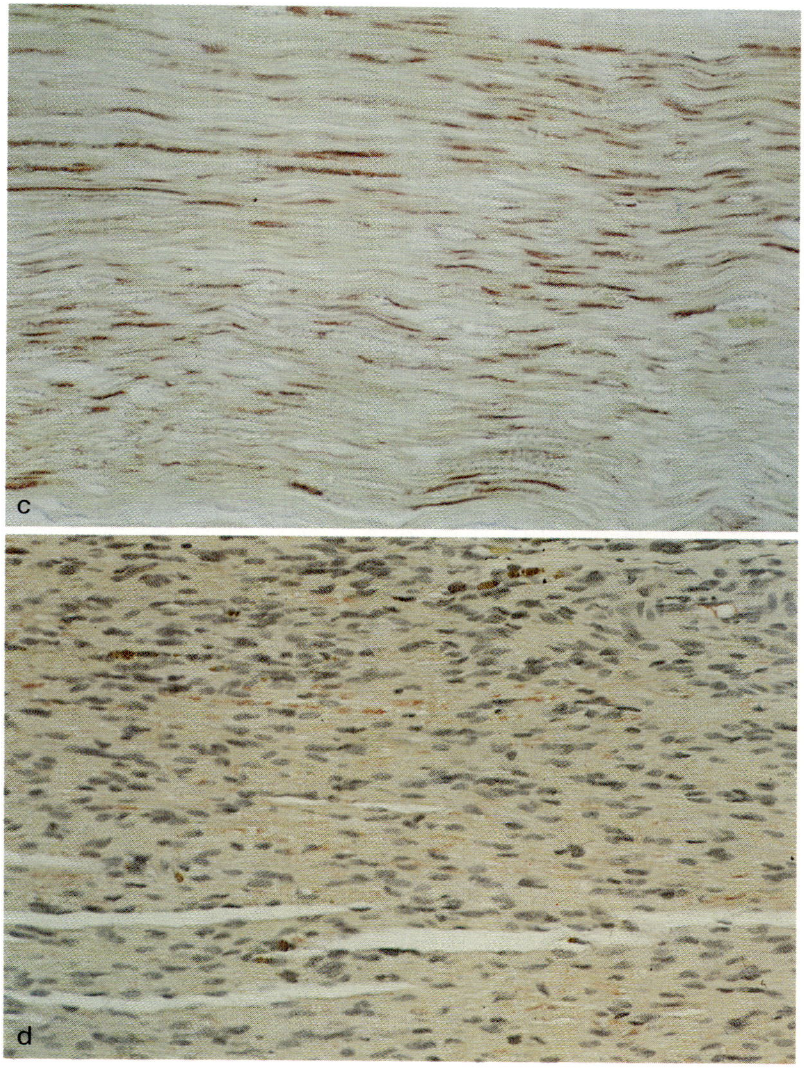

Fig. 5 c–d.

and FS groups (Fig. 5a, b, c). Significantly better regeneration of the fibers was obtained in the group FS ($p < 0.05$) (Table 1). By contrast, only a few regenerated fibers were poorly oriented in the group SUT (Fig. 5d).

Discussion

In the present long-term investigation, the morphological results indicate that local application of the biodegradable FS matrix may be beneficial for axonal regeneration. In the rat model, functional restoration may be improved after

Table 1. Orientation and regeneration of regenerated nerve fibers

	Orientation			Regeneration		
	(–)	(+)	(++)	(–)	(+)	(++)
Suture	1	3	0	0	4	0
FS	0	1	3	0	0	4*
FS + NGF	0	1	3	0	2	2

Values are scores from histological specimens evaluated blindly ($n = 4$).
–, Reflects bad orientation or regeneration; + and ++ represent intermediate or good orientation or regeneration, respectively, FS fibrin sealant; NGF, nerve growth factor
* $p<0.05$

3 months in the presence of the FS matrix enriched with exogenous NGF following sciatic nerve transection.

Following transection of the sciatic nerves, the neuritic sprouts grow from the proximal nerve across the zone of injury towards the distal segment. This is a critical moment in the regenerative process, which to a great extent determines success or failure [13].

One of the components of the fibrin matrix is fibronectin, which is also found in the extracellular matrix. The latter has been previously demonstrated to contribute the cue that stimulates and guides regenerating nerve fibers in vivo and in vitro [14, 15]. Similarly, as a basic matrix component of granulation tissue, fibrin itself serves as a temporary supporting framework for the formation of the growth cone, which is very important for the initial neuritic outgrowth [16–18]. A positive influence of the FS matrix has been previously confirmed in our short-term study, by the results of the pinch reflex test. We showed that regeneration of the leading sensory fibers was significantly faster in both fibrin matrix (FS, NGF-FS) groups than in the SUT group [9]. Furthermore, the preliminary data from the in vitro assay of neuronal cell cultures indicate that peripheral neurons survive and develop a network of neurites on the FS matrix at least as well as on the standard poly-D-lysine substratum (data not published). In the present long-term study, this finding was confirmed by the morphological data from the late phase of nerve regeneration (at 3 months after transection), where the axons were visualized by specific immunohistochemical staining with a monoclonal anti-neurofilament antibody and evaluated in a semiquantitative fashion (Fig. 5, Table 1).

It is well known that NGF mainly affects the sympathetic and sensory nerve systems. The sciatic nerve, which contains axons of motor, sympathetic and sensory neurons, is also known to be one of the pathways of NGF transport [1–7]. Both functional parameters in the present study, the serial walking-track analysis and the RMA demonstrate the recovery processes that occur in the walking behavior of the rat hind limb and the reinnervation of the corresponding muscle (TA), which are probably based on restoration of both sensory and motor functions following sciatic nerve transection. The progress of sensory restoration might improve motor functional recovery in two ways: by avoiding the complications following loss of sensory function and by indirectly inducing the motoneurons to sprout due to the activities of sensory and sympathetic neurons in transmitting messages [19–22].

References

1. Levi-Montalcini R (1987) The nerve growth factor 35 years later. Science 237: 1154–1162
2. Thoenen H, Edgar D (1985) Neurotrophic factor. Science 229: 238–242
3. Wayne DB, Heaton MB (1988) Retrograde transport of NGF by early chick embryo spinal cord motoneurons. Dev Biol 127: 220–223
4. Wood SJ, Pritchard J, Sofroniew MV (1990) Reexpression of nerve growth factor receptor after axonal injury recapitulates a developmental event in motor neurons: differential regulation when regeneration is allowed or prevented. Eur J Neurosci 2: 650–657
5. Heumann R, Korsching S, Bandtlow C, Thoenen H (1987) Changes of nerve growth factor synthesis in nonneuronal cells in response to sciatic nerve transection. J Cell Biol 104: 1623–1631
6. Heumann R, Lindholm D, Bandtlow C, Meyer M, Radeke MJ, Misko TP, Shooter E, Thoenen H (1987) Differential regulation of mRNA encoding nerve growth factor and its receptor in rat sciatic nerve during development, degeneration, and regeneration: role of macrophage. Proc Natl Acad Sci USA 84: 8735–8739
7. Raivich G, Kreutzberg GW (1987) Expression of growth factor receptors in injured nervous tissue. I. Axotomy leads to a shift in the cellular distribution of specific B-nerve growth factor binding in the injured and regenerating PNS. J Neurocytol 16: 689–700
8. Schlag G, Redl H (1988) Fibrin sealant in orthopedic surgery. Clin Orthop 27: 269–285
9. Zeng L, Worseg A, Redl H, Schlag G (1992) An experimental study of peripheral nerve repair with nerve growth factor and fibrin sealant matrix. Österreichische Gesellschaft für Plastik, Ästhetische und Rekonstruktive Chirurgie: 30th Annual Meeting, Vienna, 15–17 Oct 1992 (abstr)
10. Zeng L, Leichtfried G, Öhlinger W, Dinges HP, Redl H, Schlag G (1994) An experimental study of peripheral nerve repair with a biodegradable neurotropic and neurotrophic matrix. J Reconstr Microsurg (in press)
11. Hare GMT, Evans PJ, Mackinnon SE, Best TJ, Bain JR, Szalai JP, Hunter DA (1992) Walking track analysis: a long-term assessment of peripheral nerve recovery. Plast Reconstr Surg 89: 251–258
12. Bain JR, Mackinnon SE, Hudson AR, Falk RE, Falk JA, Hunter DA (1988) The peripheral nerve allograft: an assessment of regeneration across nerve allografts in rats immunosuppressed with cyclosporin A. Plast Reconstr Surg 82: 1052–1064
13. Lundborg G (1987) Nerve regeneration and repair. A review. Acta Orthop Scand 58: 145–169
14. Davis GE, Blaker SN, Engvall E, Varon S, Manthorpe M, Gage FH (1987) Human amnion membrane serves as a substratum for growing axons in vitro and in vivo. Science 236: 1106–1109
15. Danielsen N, Muller H, Pettmann B, Williams LR, Davis GE, Engvall E, Manthorpe M, Varon S (1988) Rat amnion membrane matrix as a substratum for regenerating axons from peripheral and central neurons: effects in a silicone chamber model. Brain Res 467: 39–50
16. Weiss P (1941) Nerve patterns: the mechanics of nerve growth. Growth, Third Growth Symposium 5: 163–203
17. Purves D (1982) Guidance of axons during development and after nerve injury. In: Nicholls JG (ed) Repair and regeneration of the nervous system. Springer, Berlin Heidelberg New York, pp 107–125

18. Willard M, Skene JHP (1982) Molecular events in axonal regeneration. In: Nicholls JG (ed) Repair and regeneration of the nervous system. Springer, Berlin Heidelberg New York, pp 71–89
19. Mackinnon SE, Dellon AL (1988) Physiology of the peripheral nerve. In: Machinnon SE, Dellon AL (eds) Surgery of the peripheral nerve. Thieme, New York, pp 11–33
20. Tomaselli KJ, Reichardt LF (1988) Peripheral motoneuron interactions with laminin and schwann cell-derived neurite-promoting molecules: developmental regulation of laminin receptor function. J Neurosci Res 21: 275–285
21. Schmidt FO, Dev P, Smith BH (1976) Electronic processing of information by brain cells. Science 193: 114–120
22. Lu B, Buck CR, Dreyfus CF, Black IB (1989) Expression of NGF and NGF receptor mRNAs in the developing brain: evidence of local delivery and action of NGF. Exp Neurol 104: 191–199

Fibrin Sealant Conduits in Peripheral Nerve Repair

N. NICOLI ALDINI, M. FINI, G. GIAVARESI, M. ROCCA, and R. GIARDINO

Abstract

A fibrin sealant sleeve treated with 2.5% glutaraldehyde to delay in vivo resorption was investigated as a conduit for nerve repair. In six Sprague-Dawley rats the ischiatic nerve was transected to obtain a 1 cm gap, which was bridged by grafting the conduit between the proximal and distal ends. The surgical procedure was performed under general anesthesia using a micro surgical technique. Controls at 3 and 6 months demonstrated a recovery of electrical properties of the nerve and morphological evidence of axonal regeneration through the lumen of the conduit. The wall of the conduit was easily recognizable in every case. These results confirm that the conduit is effective as a nerve prosthesis. Our preliminary results, confirming that sealant properties are lost, show that the degradation of Tissucol is modified by glutaraldehyde treatment.

Introduction

Autologous nerve grafts are the most common surgical procedure when peripheral nerve reconstruction is required and there is a defect between the proximal and distal stump of the nerve trunk. Nevertheless, the capability of axons to regenerate through various types of conduits placed between the proximal and distal segments of the nerve suggests that such devices may present alternatives to autografts. The ideal nerve conduit is easily available, biodegradable and poorly antigenic [1].

In our Experimental Surgery Laboratory, research was performed on conduits made of biological or degradable materials [2, 3].

The literature [4] and our personal experience [5] emphasize the biocompatibility of fibrin sealant. Since it has been used in nerve coaptation with satisfactory results [6, 7], we evaluated the feasibility, employing this material derived from a regeneration chamber, of its use as a prosthesis in nerve repair.

The following questions were examined:

1. Is it possible, using fibrin glue, to make a conduit with an inner diameter of 1–2 mm?

2. Since the in vivo resorption rate of fibrin glue (7–14 g) is less than required of a guide for nerve regeneration, is it possible to delay the degradation of the material?
3. Is the conduit obtained in this way suitable for peripheral nerve grafting?
4. When grafted, is the conduit effective in allowing nerve regeneration into its lumen?

The animal model in which these investigations were performed was adjusted according to the guidelines of the International Guide on Animal Biomedical Research and of the Ethical Code for Animal Experimentation of C.I.O.M.S., and of the Council Directive n. 86/609/CEE.

The nerve was explanted and fixed in 10 % buffered formalin. Longitudinal and transverse sections were stained with Hematoxylin-Eosin and by the Bodian method. Immunohistochemical investigations for axons and Schwann cells in the lumen of the conduit were also performed (Universal immunoperoxidase staining kit, Ortho Diagnostic System, Cambridge, Mass. USA).

Materials and Methods

Making the Conduit

The material employed for this purpose is the human fibrin sealant Tissucol (Immuno, Vienna), prepared by reconstituting the two components following the standard procedure using thrombin 500.

The glue was sprayed, by means of the Duploject system, on a turning Teflon 22G catheter, making a sleeve of a few centimeters. It was then placed into 2.5 % buffered glutaraldehyde for 72 h. After the treatment fibrin glue sleeves were slipped off from the catheter, carefully washed with saline solution, and cut to obtain segments of 1 cm length. The perviousness of the conduits was promptly checked under operative microscope, and those that presented faults or breaks in the wall were discarded. The selected conduits were stored in 40 % ethanol until implantation.

The final product was a tube of soft consistence and fairly crumbly, but strong enough to be crossed by suture threads without excessive damage (Fig. 1).

The Animal Model

The conduits were implanted in six male Sprague-Dawley rats under general anesthesia induced with chloralium hydrate (1 ml/100 g weight intraperitoneally). The ischiatic nerve was exposed at the thigh through the gluteus muscle and transected above the tibioperoneal bifurcation; a segment was excised to obtain an 8 mm gap. The nerve was then repaired by grafting the conduit between the two stumps; it was sutured proximally and distally to the epineurium with two 10/0 nylon stitches. Each procedure was performed bilaterally, with magnification (Fig. 2).

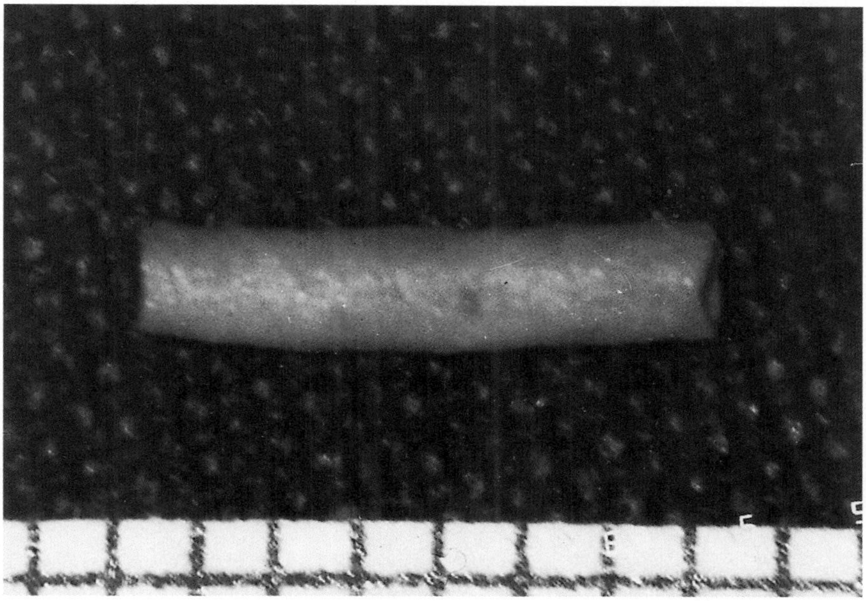

Fig. 1. The fibrin sealant glutaraldehyde treated conduit (operative microscope)

At the end of the intervention the animals were housed in single cages and received food and water ad libitum.

Controls were performed after 3 and 6 months. Under general anesthesia, induced as previously described, the nerve was carefully dissected at the part including the conduit. EMG controls were performed stimulating the nerve above the prosthesis and recording the evoked potential on flexor superficialis digitorum muscle.

Results

All the animals survived without complications, except for trophic plantar ulcers that appeared during the first few weeks and healed in 3–4 months. In all the rats, at surgical reexploration the conduit was easily recognizable, of yellowish color and surrounded by a vascularized connective cuff.

Evoked muscle action potentials were recorded after stimulation of the nerve trunk, showing a recovery of conduction already after 3 months. After 6 months, the electrophysiological pattern was similar to that of normal ischiatic nerve.

A transverse section in the mid-portion of the conduit (Fig. 3) demonstrated that its wall was readily detectable and the lumen was filled by newly formed tissue, divided from the inside surface by a thin space. In the histological sections stained with hematoxylin-eosin, the wall appeared homogeneously eosinophilic; a foreign body reaction was present, surrounding the

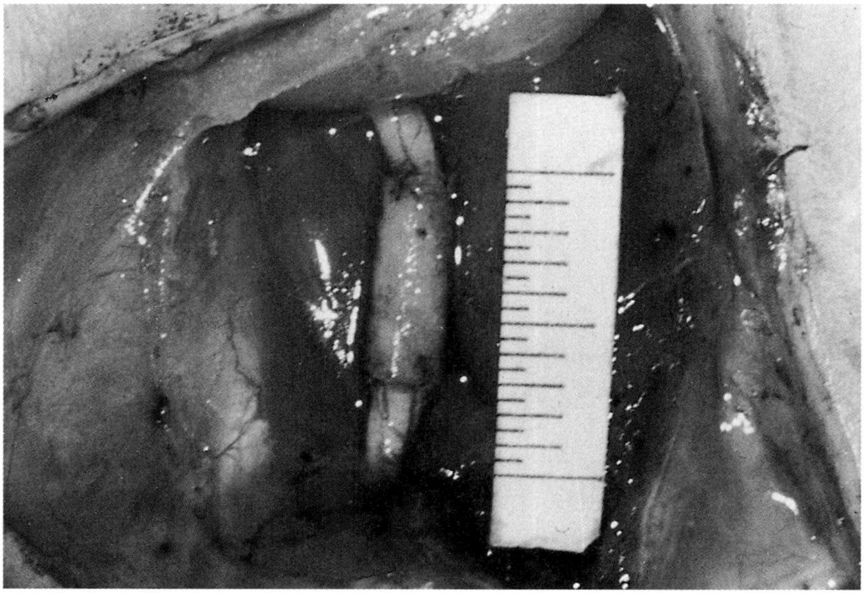

Fig. 2. The conduit after the grafting between the two stumps of the transected ischiatic nerve (operative microscope)

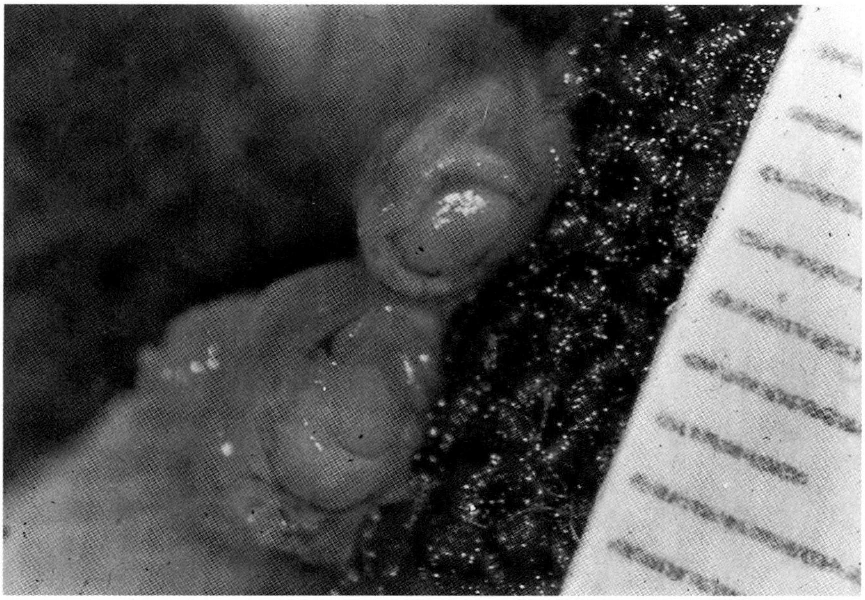

Fig. 3. A section in the midportion of the conduit, 6 months after grafting: the wall is easily detectable and the lumen is filled by newly formed tissue (operative microscope)

sutures. The tissue in the lumen reunites the two stumps of the interrupted nerve; longitudinally oriented argyrophilic fibers were present. Immuno histochemical investigations for axons and Schwann cells were positive.

Discussion

On the basis of these preliminary results, we conclude that:

1. Fibrin glue can be used in making tubular devices; the procedure is rather simple even if the conduit is made by hand. The method can be improved using more exact procedures, to standardize the characteristics of the conduit. Treatment with glutaraldehyde strengthens and stabilizes the material compared to untreated fibrin glue, imparting to the conduit a better maneuvrability during the intervention.

2. A conduit employed as a regeneration chamber should not be reabsorbed before 4–6 months to permit reorganization of regenerating tissue. This assumption is in accord with the literature regarding degradable conduits [8] and fulfills the biologic prerequisites of the regeneration chamber. The in vivo resorption rate of fibrin glue is underneath these conditions, requiring 7–14 days. For this reason we have evaluated a procedure of chemical denaturation to preserve the material from enzymatic attack and have applied, for this purpose, a method previously described by Yannas [9]: treatment with glutaraldehyde of protein-containing substrates is effective in slowing down their in vivo degradation. Our results confirm this assumption, as the conduit was still recognizeable 6 months after the implant. Until now, however, it has not been possible to establish if the conduit is or is not eventually completely degradable and what is the time of resorption.

3. The structural features and mechanical properties of the conduit make it compatible with use in peripheral nerve reconstruction. Nevertheless, it is necessary to point out that the resistance of the wall to the stress arising when it is crossed by the stitches is rather small and it is easy to damage the wall with the sutures. This problem may be solved by also using the sealant to fasten the conduit to the nerve stumps.

4. Functional and morphological data confirm that transected ischiatic nerve is able to regenerate through the lumen of the conduit, bridging an 8 mm gap with recovery of electrical properties. However, a more extensive follow-up is required to evaluate, over a longer time, the organization of the regenerating nerve. Up to this point, it is only possible to state that the fibrin sealant conduit acts as a guide allowing reunion of the nerve stumps and serving as a regeneration chamber.

The data collected until now permit us to draw some conclusions and some plans to develop our research: Fibrin sealant is useful for making tubular devices suitable for particular surgical needs. Applied in nerve reconstruction, these devices allow axonal regeneration into their lumen. It is possible to chemically modify the fibrin glue, to condition its resorption in vivo; nevertheless we do not know if glutaraldehyde is the sole compound appropriate for this purpose. Other methods of treatment may give the conduit better mechanical properties. The time needed for the conduits resorption, in our experience, is over 6 months, providing a lapse of time adequate to allow nerve regeneration in experimental animals.

Acknowledgement. Financial support of this research by Istituti Ortopedici Rizzoli, Ricerca Corrente, area n. 2, is gratefully acknowledged.

References

1. Mackinnon SE (1989) Surgical management of the peripheral nerve gap. Clin Plast Surg 16 (3): 587–603
2. Nicoli Aldini N, Stea S, Rocca M, Giardino R, Poppi V, Pizzoferrato A (1990) PTEE versus biological prostheses to bridge a nerve gap: experimental evaluation. Int J Artif Organs 13 (9): 625
3. Nicoli Aldini N, Stea S, Righini S, Rocca M, Fini M, Govoni D, Giardino R, Pizzoferrato A (1991) Nerve regeneration through biological prosthesis. Int J Artif Organs 14 (9): 586
4. Schlag G, Redl H (1989) Fibrin sealant: efficacy, quality and safety. In: Waclawiczek HW (ed) Progress in fibrin sealing. Springer, Berlin Heidelberg New York, pp 3–17
5. Giardino R (1985) I collanti biologici e artificiali. In: Marrano D (ed) Attualità sul trattamento delle ferite, piaghe, ulcere. Monduzzi, Bologna, pp 11–16
6. Moy OL, Peimer CA, Koniuch MP (1988) Fibrin sealant adhesive versus nonabsorbable microsuture in peripheral nerve repair. J Hand Surg 13A: 273–279
7. Maragh H, Meyer BS, Davenport D, Gould JD, Terzis JK (1990) Morphofunctional evaluation of fibrin glue versus microsuture nerve repairs. J Reconstr Microsurg 6 (4): 331–337
8. Keeley RD, Nguyen KD, Stephanides MJ, Padilla J, Rosen JM (1991) The artificial nerve graft: a comparison of blended elastomer-hydrogel with polyglycoli acid conduits. J Reconstr Microsurg 7 (2): 93–100
9. Yannas IV, Norregard TV, Silver J, Zervas NT, Krik JF, Colt MJ (1987) Relations between properties of collagen-glycosaminoglycan graft and morphology of regenerating nerve. Transactions of the 13th Annual Meeting of the Society for Biomaterials, June 3–7, 1987, New York

Ten Years' Experience Using Tissucol in the Repair of the Brachial Plexus and Neighboring Nerves

A. O. Narakas[1] † and C. Bonnard

Abstract

During a 10 year period, starting in November 1980, a cylindrical tube of clotted plasma was used in 218 patients to join the trimmed stumps of 549 trunks, cords and nerves forming the brachial plexus or lying close to it, e.g., the spinal accessory nerve. Reconstruction was obtained by direct neurorrhaphy in a few cases and by neurotization and/or by autologous grafts in the vast majority of instances. The classical technique of interfascicular repair was slightly modified in order to diminish the quantity of connective tissue at the apposition site between the central and the peripheral stump. Whenever necessary 9/0 to 11/0 nylon superficial stay sutures were used to reinforce the junction. Muscular power was evaluated in 200 patients. The average age was 25.6 years and the average follow-up 15.14 months. Repair of spinal nerves, trunks and cords yielded. In 64 % of the patients the results were better than M2+, according to the Highet (MRC) score. Neurotization using the spinal accessory nerve and other cervical motor rami led to positive results in 75 % of the patients while only 57 % of the patients who underwent intercostal nerve repair improved. By contrast, 84 % of fair to good results with repair of various nerves close to the plexus, repair of the median and ulnar nerves being the least successful. Although a comparison between suturing and gluing was made, in such complex surgery it is not possible to demonstrate statistically the superiority of one method over the other. There was certainly a gain in operation time, and the sprouts crossed the junction's interface more easily so the total regeneration time was a little shorter. The quality of results are, however, the same after adequate follow-up. The reduction of failures witnessed when using fibrin sealant probably has to be attributed to the experience both surgeons involved in the study have gained during the additional 10 years of nerve repair.

Introduction

In the late 1960s, while visiting Great Britain, one of us (AN) saw that the fibrin clot method of Seddon [1] was still being used on rare occasions. The technique was said to not be very practical or reliable, and it looked less precise

1 Deceased on November 25th, 1993

than the microsurgical fascicular or fascicular group repair already introduced worldwide [2–7]. Participating in a brachial plexus symposium in Lausanne, Kuderna [8] demonstrated, as early as 1975, an improved fibrin sealant that produced almost perfect junctions. It took us, however, 4 years to overcome the prejudice against fibrin glue. Dr. Narakas started to use it, in the second half of 1979, for repair of peripheral nerves, introducing it for plexus repair in November of that year. In the beginning he applied it in every fifth patient. After registering the first favorable results, in the summer of 1980, Tissucol was adopted for neurosynthesis in every other case and from June 1981 it was used systematically in every instance.

This study concerns patients operated on by the authors only, either together or independently using the same techniques.

Methods

Tissucol

During the 10-years period of the survey the method for using Tissucol has varied. Initially 500 units of thrombin (NIH-U) and 3000 KIU/ml of aprotinin were applied. Later on, the fibrinolysis inhibitor was diminished to 300 and even to 100 KIU/ml to be increased again to 1000 in 1985, as it was learned that amounts of that order would not produce fibrosis while still ensuring stability and acceptable strength of repair. The preparation of grafts underwent also some changes; however, in the last 8 years it has hardly been modified. The steps of sealing with fibrin are described here in detail, as there are some differences when repairing big paucifascicular trunks or multifascicular nerves. In order to diminish the amount of fibrous tissue which impedes sprouts crossing the repair site, we isolated the individual fascicles inside the ends of the grafts, trimming them in a special way. They were cleaned from adventitial and epineural tissue, over a distance of 5–8 mm, with a very sharp ophthalmic blade or microscissors, leaving them exposed. They were then assembled to form a tight bundle of approximatively the same diameter as the cut surface of the fascicle or the fascicular group in the nerve trunk which they had to cover. Because of resection of nonnervous tissue, grouping of more fascicles was needed to reach the required section than when using a conventional cable graft. Indeed, almost twice as many were usually required to repair a given nerve segment, e.g., six to eight grafts were needed instead of three to four, as in standard interfascicular grafting. With extensive damage, the proper amount of graft could not always be obtained, even when harvesting both sural nerves, the medial cutaneous nerve of the forearm, including sometimes the sensory branch of the radial nerve. On certain occasions supplementary grafts could be gained from nerves originating in avulsed roots, e.g., the ulnar nerve in C7, C8, T1 root avulsion. In such circumstances the epineurium would be peeled off from the harvested nerve trunk to foster its revascularization. The epineurium was maintained when the ulnar nerve was used either as a pedicled graft or a free one, which was revascularized by a microsurgical anastomosis. In such cases, and when dealing with multifascicular structures particularly in sites proximal to branching off of rami, we performed fascicular group matching: two or three grafts were assembled to bridge one fascicular group, while other cables did the same for the remaining ones. When doing so, very small quantities of Tissucol were used inside the nerve. Then a sleeve of fibrin would be created to surround the junction externally.

For trunk repair containing one or two fascicular groups, the construction of the bundle was done with grafts, each one having a slightly different length, those on the outside being longer than those in the middle. Thus a spindle-shaped cable was formed. This disposition was intended to favor revascularization of the grafts by their bed on which they were glued with one or two drops of Tissucol.

A slip about five times as wide as the diameter of the structure in repair was cut from a surgical glove and put underneath the repair site. Trimming of stumps and cable was performed immediately before performing the junction, to minimize protrusion of fibers on the cut surface. A nerve holder and a very sharp disposable blade were used, in preference to microscissors as proposed by Meyer and Smahel [9]. We exposed the freshly cut ends as little as possible to air, apposing and aligning them quickly. We did not use the Duploject in most cases, but applied the two solutions separately, drop by drop, the size of the drops being determined by the gauge of the needles. The smaller the structures to be repaired, the smaller we made the drops. The duploject was used when repairing tilted segments, to avoid flowing away of the solutions before they could mix and clot. Only a very thin, transparent layer of Tissucol was applied in order to allow inspection of the junction. Small adjustments of the fascicular alignment could be made with microforceps during the 10 or 15 s following application of the sealant. The rubber slip was wrapped around the junction and left for at least 3 min, i.e., until the glue had hardened enough to form a smooth and thin membrane. In all portions of the neck and chest where small spontaneous movements of tissues could not be avoided (e.g., caused by respiration) 9/0 to 11/0 nylon stay-stitches were used. They were easily put through the layer of Tissucol, catching on the parafascicular tissue which could not recede before the needle because the clotted glue had stabilized the apposed structures. Head, neck and shoulders were usually immobilized for 3–4 days and the upper limb was kept at rest across the chest for 3 weeks, avoiding lateral abduction in the shoulder for an additional 3 weeks so as not to stretch prematurely the repaired structures. Nevertheless, in three surgically verified instances, breaking down of the junction occurred. All three concerned direct neurotizations of the musculocutaneous nerve by intercostal nerves. In one patient a hematoma developed within 24 h after operation requiring surgical draining. In the two other patients significant vomiting or coughing was noted after surgery explaining disruption of the repair.

Assessing Repair

It is necessary to comment on the complexity of recording results of brachial plexus repair. They can be assessed to some extent using the grading Highet proposed in the 1940s to the Medical Research Council of Great Britain [10]. A functional scale, as worked up by Narakas [11] in collaboration with P. Raimondi and A. Morelli from Legnano, Italy, is more realistic. The former is simpler and evaluates the power of each muscle without depicting usefulness achieved. The latter represents a global functional approach. In this study success or lack of success of a given method of repair were to be analyzed, and it seemed that Highet's grading was sufficient for that purpose. In addition we wanted to compare our results with those from the years 1965–1980, when the MRD scale was the only grading system available for assessment. We scaled our junction to the one obtained by classical microsuturing at that time using 8/0 to 12/0 nylon. The authors and/or trained assisting surgeons or physicians performed the examinations. A rating of M0 to M2+ was considered a failure, M3– to M3+ as a fair result and M4 – to M5 as a good result. Only clearly established results are reported here.

This method is easy to apply for evaluation of a given repaired structure, provided the latter supplies an elementary function, such as ensured by the axillary nerve innervating the deltoid or the musculocutaneous nerve supplying the biceps and brachialis. No sophisticated sensory testing is required. Evaluation becomes extremely complex, however, when it concerns nerves such as the median or the ulnar which innervate many muscles. Therefore, in this study, we do not mention at all sensation resulting from repair of median and ulnar nerves close to the brachial plexus. Another reason for rejecting the complete evaluation of these nerves is the small number of such repairs that we did, rendering statistical evaluation unreliable. In addition the assessement of motor results obtained only by very proximal repair of the radial, median and ulnar nerves also has its limitations. For example, in C5–C7 repair, recovery of the brachioradialis, an elbow flexor, has to be excluded as it may paradoxically downgrade triceps function, activated not on elbow flexion with the biceps, but on extension, because of undifferentiated recovery of fibers constituting the radial nerve. Goals regarding extent of recovery have to be limited also. We averaged only the power of muscles in the forearm reinnervated by the median and ulnar nerves, neglecting the hand, as intrinsic muscle function of it will not be obtained in adult plexus reconstruction. Thus, a powerful flexion of wrist and fingers without recovery of opposition of thumb and presence of clawing was considered a good result. Accessory nerve function was evaluated in isolated injuries of that nerve which were mostly iatrogenic. They were graded good when full elevation of the shoulder and arm was obtained and the scapula was not lateralized more than 2 cm as compared to the healthy side, serratus anterior function being normal in these patients. This can be considered as ≥ 75 % of normal function. It was claimed as being fair when the upper trapezius had recovered 75 % and the middle trapezius 50 % of their function; contraction of the lower trapezius was neglected in this study. It can be evaluated only when a full range of motion is present and is considered only to establish an excellent result. However, a distinction between excellent and good was not introduced in this study.

When suprascapular nerve repair enabled abduction of the arm above 90° produced by the supraspinatus muscle alone (e.g., when the deltoid is com-

Table 1. Repair from spinal nerves, trunks, and cords (262 receivers)

Donors	Receivers (*n*)	Results (*n*)		
		Good	Fair	Poor
Accessory phrenic nerve	Long thoracic nerve (3) and (2) anteroinferior thoracic nerve	3	2	0
C5	Long thoracic nerve (3)	2	1	0
C5	Suprascapular nerve (51)	13	15	23
C5 (C6)	Lateral cords (93)	46	22	25
C5–C6	Posterior cords (82)	26	22	34
C7	Radial, median ulnar nerves (22)	6	7	9
C8–T1	Median, ulnar nerves (6)	0	3	3
Total (%)		96 (37)	72 (27)	94 (36)

pletely paralyzed in neurotizations for avulsions of C5, C6–C7 and more), the result was considered as being better than M3+, i.c., good. An abduction from 40° to 80° was considered as fair. When an external rotation to the sagittal plane was achieved it was graded as 3–, i.e., fair; beyond that limit it deserved the qualification of good. Both MRC gradings were added and divided by two to obtain an average of suprascapular nerve function. Concerning the posterior cord or radial nerve function a result was estimated as being not better than fair when finger extension by the long forearm extensors was not recovered, while triceps and wrist extensor function were regained. When, in addition to that, metacarpophalangeal long finger extension almost to 0° and an acceptable thumb IP joint extension and abduction was obtained the result was said to be good.

The following anatomical segments were considered. Repair from spinal nerves or primary trunks means that the stumps of the anterior branches of spinal nerves C5 to T1 or the upper, middle and/or lower trunk were connected directly or by grafts to their distal counterparts. Repair of cords was also included in this group, as most of the time traction lesions extended from one

Table 2. Repair from spinal accessory nerve (XI) and deep cervical plexus

Receivers (*n*)	Results (*n*)		
	Good	Fair	Poor
Suprascapular nerve (53)	13	29	10
Posterior cords (5)	1	2	2
Musculocutaneous nerve (7)	2	2	3
Avulsed C7 (1)	0	1	0
Long thoracic nerve (7)	2	2	3
Anteroinferior thoracic nerves for lower pectoralis major (1)	1	0	0
Total (%)	19 (26)	36 (49)	18 (25)

Table 3. Neurotization with intercostal nerves

	Results (*n*)		
Receivers (*n*)	Good	Fair	Poor
Axillary nerve (2)	0	1	1
Anteroinferior thoracic nerve for inferior pectoralis major (15)	7	4	4
Musculocutaneous nerve (39)	7	15	17
Posterior cords (4)	0	2	2
Median, ulnar nerves (10)	1	3	6
Total (%)	15 (21)	25 (36)	30 (43)

anatomical structure to the next. Table 1 shows what was obtained at different levels using different donors. For neurotization a direct neurorrhaphy was generally performed while repair of other segments implied autologous nerve grafting. Table 2 refers to the use of the spinal accessory nerve and motor rami of the deep cervical plexus as a source of axon sprouts. In four patients intermediate autologous grafts were used.

Table 3 refers to neurotization with intercostal nerves. Quite often the upper ones, i.e., T3–T5, were connected directly to the receivers, while small grafts were required when using T6–T7. Finally, there were repairs of nerve trunks in the neighborhood of the plexus, such as the axillary, the musculocutaneous and others. The results are shown in Table 4. All patients had a follow-up of at least 2 years.

Table 4. Repair of nerve trunks

	Results (*n*)		
Nerves repaired (*n*)	Good	Fair	Poor
Spinal accessory nerves (15)	7	7	1
Suprascapular nerves (10)	3	5	2
Grafts from suprascapular nerve to supraspinatus muscle (2) and direct intramuscular implantations (2)	1	1	2
Thoracodorsal nerve transfers onto the axillary nerve (4)	0	3	1
Axillary nerves (57)	39	16	2
Musculocutaneous nerves (28)	18	7	3
Radial nerves (11)	5	2	4
Median nerves (8)	1	2	5
Ulnar nerves (7)	2	2	3
Total (%)	76 (53)	45 (31)	23 (16)

Results

As Table 1 shows, the very small accessory phrenic nerve is a quite potent donor and reinnervates well such voluminous muscles as the pectoralis major or serratus anterior. It was connected directly to one of the rami constituting the long thoracic nerve. It was usually completely paralyzed in avulsions concerning the three upper and higher roots. Reconstruction of the suprascapular nerve from C5 yields a good result only when the proximal stump of C5 is quite long. The positive results (55 %) are not as numerous when using a healthy nerve as a neurotizer, like the spinal accessory (Table 2, 81 %). This shows once again that in stretch injuries damage ascends quite high in the proximal portion of the affected structure so that repair is performed not from entirely healthy fascicles. Repair of lateral and posterior cords yields satisfactory results (Table 1, 66 %) because mostly proximal muscles, such as pectoralis major, biceps, brachialis, triceps, wrist extensors, are tested for evaluation. In lateral cord repairs some axon sprouts will travel down the contribution for the median nerve; their regeneration is difficult to assess because their functional recovery will be masked by the fiber activity coming from the normal lower roots, i.e., a good flexor ulnaris and pronator quadratus will compensate weakness of the flexor carpi radialis and pronator teres. By contrast repair of the median and ulnar nerves from C7, C8 and T1 will yield a much poorer result. The radial nerve behaves far better in this respect; its repair sometimes yields a good result and compensation by musculotendinous transfers is easy when the median and ulnar nerves are functional.

The spinal accessory nerve is a very potent neurotizer. It receives contributions from the cervical ansae, one of them joining the nerve at the level of the clavicle 1–2 cm below the branching off of the rami for the upper trapezius. When the XIth is transected distal to those rami and proximal to the contribution from the cervical ansa, at least two thirds of the function of the trapezius muscle are retained. The loss of one third is unimportant for the function of the shoulder which is anyway limited in these cases.

In the vast majority of the patients the XIth nerve is directly connected to the suprascapular nerve. It is difficult to regain a more or less normal function; only more often, abduction and, rarely, a good external rotation are recovered, the infraspinatus remaining poor. More distant nerves cannot be connected directly to the XIth. They require an intermediate graft, thus downgrading the results by approximately 30 %.

Rami of the deep cervical plexus are very useful to restore function of the long thoracic nerve, which is important for the control of scapulothoracic motion. They can also be used to neurotize anterior thoracic nerves in order to reconstruct adduction of the arm by pectoralis major. We often neurotize them with an upper intercostal nerve (Table 3).

In our hands intercostal nerve transfers have not yielded as good results as those obtained by the Japanese surgeons [12, 13], who claim in children and young adults a success rate of 82 %. While intercostobrachial neurotization is quite satisfactory, it does not seem very useful to attempt to reanimate the median or ulnar nerve with intercostal nerves. They present functions too complex to be monitored by such primitive nerves as intercostals. Possibly a transfer onto motor rami well selected in forearm muscles using a long intermediate graft would be a more sensible approach.

Direct axillary and muscolocutaneous repairs, which are performed in the vast majority of cases by grafting, yield quite good results. A favorable outcome was obtained in 94 % of repairs. The global results in Table 4 are severely downgraded by the modest percentage (54 %) of positive results obtained when repairing the radial, medial and ulnar nerves close to the brachial plexus. Paradoxically repair of fascicles of these nerves in the proximal portion of the plexus does not seem to give results different from those obtained by a more distal repair (Tables 1, 4).

Repair of the spinal accessory nerve has yielded good results for many years [14]. It is far easier to reconstruct by gluing than by suturing the small grafts, some being local sensory rami of the cervical plexus that retain partially their vascular connections. The significantly better results obtained gluing them and adding one or two superficial sutures compared to only suturing them (93 % vs 71 %) reflects only partially the superiority of gluing small caliber nerves. The remaining part can be explained by the better experience of the authors in their repair and handling of the nerve which has often been used in neurotizations over the last 12 years. Identification of the distal stump of the XIth is not always easy, and errors in that respect can explain some of the failures in the past. Some of the repairs performed by suturing were done after long delays, up to 3 years between injury and reconstruction. The deleterious role of such a long interval has been well documented [15].

Discussion

Already in 1942, Seddon and Medawar [1] were saying that it was probable that plasma will prove to be of great value in primary suture of divided nerves and that it should be used for repair of large defects by grafting in preference to all other materials. Improvements in the homogeneity of fibrin glue and the ease of application even in an awkward position has facilitated its handling, rendering less strenuous maintenance of fascicular alignment and shortening the time of operation. Can it improve the results compared to the use of microsutures? Mechanical factors acting at the junction site cannot increase axon synthesis by the neurone and accelerate regeneration. Therefore, the only possible improvement is quicker crossing of sprouts at the junction, as already noted by Young and Medawar [16]. They found in rabbits a gain of 1 day, which is not significant. In our hands, glue fostered the crossing of a sufficient number of fibers to elicit function, the gain being approximately 2 months. The sealant is not an obstacle for sprout progression, unlike stitches, which significantly deviate the direction of fiber growth causing malalignment. We had one almost experimental proof of extremely satisfactory outgrowth of sprouts after grafting a sciatic nerve in a patient in whom we had excised an apparently benign tumor. It was in fact highly malignant and an exarticulation at the hip was performed 10 days later, histology showing an almost complete resorption of Tissucol and beautiful regeneration cones with little distorsion of fibers.

Table 5. Comparison between results obtained by suturing vs by gluing

Nerve	Results (*n*) and percentages Good		Fair		Poor or nil	
Spinal accessory						
Suturing	5		5		4	
Gluing	7		7		1	
Axillary						
Suturing	15	83 %	0	0 %	3	7 %
Gluing	35	64 %	18	33 %	2	3 %
Musculocutaneous						
Suturing	8	67 %	3	25 %	1	8 %
Gluing	21	66 %	8	25 %	3	9 %
Radial						
Suturing	1	17 %	4	67 %	1	17 %
Gluing	5	45 %	2	18 %	4	36 %
Total						
Suturing	29	68 %	12	24 %	9	18 %
Gluing	68	60 %	35	31 %	10	9 %

Late controls of nerves sutured or glued showed, however, similar results (Table 5), the sutured ones catching up after 3–1 years [17]: 93 % favorable results vs 92 %. Thus the two methods are equivalent. The smaller number of good results (60 % vs 68 %) can be explained by the longer follow-up in the sutured series, as it was seen in many instances that results continued to improve between the fifth and ninth year after a successful brachial plexus repair. The reduction of failures by 50 % in the glued series can be attributed to the increased skill and experience of the authors.

References

1. Seddon HJ, Medawar PB (1942) Fibrin suture of human nerves. Lancet II: 87–88
2. Edshage S (1964) Peripheral nerve suture. A technique for improved intraneural topography. Acta Chir Scand Suppl 331: 1–104
3. Kurze T (1964) Microtechniques in neurological surgery. Clin Neurosurg 11: 128–137
4. Michon J, Masse P (1964) Le moment optimum de la suture nérveuse dans les plaies du membre supérieur. Rev Chir Orthop 50: 205–212
5. Smith JW (1964) Microsurgery of peripheral nerves. Plast Reconstr Surg 33: 317–329
6. Millesi H, Ganglberger J, Berger A (1966) Erfahrungen mit der Mikrochirurgie peripherer Nerven. Langenbecks Arch Klin Chir 316: 723–727
7. Bora FW (1967) Peripheral nerve repair in cats. The fascicular stitch. J Bone Joint Surg 49-A: 659–666
8. Kuderna M, Dinges M, Redl H (1980) Die Fibrinklebung in der Mikrochirurgie der peripheren Nerven. Hefte Unfallheilkd 148: 822–825
9. Meyer VE, Smahel J (1980) The surgical cut-surface of peripheral nerves. Int J Microsurg 2: 187–192
10. Zachary RB (1954) Results of nerve suture. In: Seddon HJ (ed) Peripheral nerve injuries. HMSO, London, p 355 (Medical Research Council Report Series)

11. Narakas AO (1988) Repair of brachial plexus trunks. In: Brunelli G (ed) Textbook of Microsurgery. Masson, Paris, pp 751–758
12. Nagano A, Tsuyama N, Ochiai N, Hara T, Takahashi M (1989) Direct nerve crossing with the intercostal nerve to treat avulsion injuries of the brachial plexus. J Hand Surg 14A: 980–985
13. Doi K, Sakai K, Kuwata N, Ihara K, Kawai S (1991) Reconstruction of finger and elbow function after complete avulsion of the brachial plexus. J Hand Surg 16A: 796–803
14. Harris HH, Dickey JR (1965) Nerve grafting to restore function of the trapezius muscle after radical neck dissection (a preliminary report). Ann Otol Rhinol Laryngol 74: 880–886
15. Hentz VR, Narakas A (1988) The results of microsurgical reconstruction in complete brachial plexus palsy. Assessing outcome and predicting results. Orthop Clin North Am 19: 107–114
16. Young JZ, Medawar PB (1940) Fibrin suture of peripheral nerves. Measurement of the rate of regeneration. Lancet II: 126–128
17. Narakas A (1988) The use of fibrin glue in repair of peripheral nerves. Orthop Clin North Am 19: 187–199

Fibrin Glue Anastomosis of the Facial Nerve

O. Sterkers, N. Julien, D. Bouccara, and J. M. Sterkers

Abstract

The facial nerve was repaired by fibrin glue anastomosis in the cerebellopontine angle, the petrous bone and/or the parotid in 70 patients. End-to-end (n = 22) or cable graft (n = 32) anastomosis of the facial nerve or hypoglosso-facial anastomosis (n = 16) was performed for 49 cerebellopontine angle tumors (45 acoustic neuromas and four meningiomas), 13 petrous bone tumors (nine facial neuromas, two cholesteatomas, one papillary epithelial tumor, one hemangioma) five petrous bone fractures, one parotid gland tumor with petrous extension and for two patients with iatrogenic intraparotid section of the nerve trunk. Grade III facial regeneration was observed in 62 % of the patients, followed for at least 1 year. End-to-end and cable graft anastomoses in the cerebellopontine angle, in the petrous bone and in the parotid led to 59 % and 65 % grade III regeneration, respectively. Grade III and grade IV regeneration was observed in 50 % of the patients after hypoglosso-facial anastomosis. We include that fibrin glue provides a safe technique for facial nerve repair. The anastomosis should be performed without tension and vascularization of the nerve should be preserved.

Introduction

Since the application of fibrin glue in otology and neuro-otology, new techniques for grafting the facial nerve have been developed [1–3]. Fibrin glue has been shown to be a suitable, simple, and rapid method for the anastomosis of nerve endings. In a previous report of 56 patients [3], we demonstrated the usefulness of fibrin glue in the anastomosis of the facial nerve in the cerebellopontine angle (CPA), the petrous bone or extracranially in the parotid gland. The fibrin glued anastomosis of the facial nerve gave good results whether a cable graft was performed or not.

Table 1. Etiology and localization of the facial nerve anastomosis (n = 70)

Site	Etiology	n
CPA and IAC	Acoustic neuroma	45
	Meningioma	4
Petrous bone	Facial nerve neuroma	9
	Cholesteatoma	2
	Epithelial tumor	1
	Hemangioma	1
	Fracture	5
Parotid gland	Iatrogenic section	2
	Cylindroma	1

Material and Methods

A total of 70 patients with facial palsy due to a section of the facial nerve were studied (Table 1). In 70 %, a tumor had developed in the CPA and the internal auditory canal (IAC). In 26 %, a tumor or a fracture involved the petrous bone. In the remaining 4 %, the facial nerve trunk was sectioned or invaded by the tumor extracranially in the parotid gland. A termino-terminal anastomosis, sometimes with a rerouting of the facial nerve within the petrous bone was performed, in 31 %. A cable graft anastomosis, using in most cases a sample of the great auricular nerve or in other rare cases the sural nerve, was done in 46 %. A hypoglosso-facial anastomosis was performed in 23 %. Anastomoses were usually done with Tissucol (Immuno, France); in two patients, an autologous fibrin glue was used. The same protocol was used in all patients, a few millimeters of the epineural sheet were removed except in the CPA or IAC segments of the nerve, which are devoid of epineurium; the nerve trunk was sectioned perpendiculary with a knife; in the petrous bone and in the parotid gland, the internal part of the fallopian canal and the gland itself, respectively, were used as a support for the anastomosis; in the CPA, a lyophilized sheet of dura was used as an anastomosis support when necessary. A traction between the nerve endings was avoided and a cable graft was performed if a residual traction between the nerve endings was noticed. The results were expressed following the grading scale of House and Brackmann [4] (Table 2).

Table 2. House and Brackmann grading of facial function

Grade	Function level
I	Normal
II	Mild dysfunction
III	Moderate dysfunction
IV	Moderately severe dysfunction
V	Severe dysfunction
VI	Total paralysis

From [4].

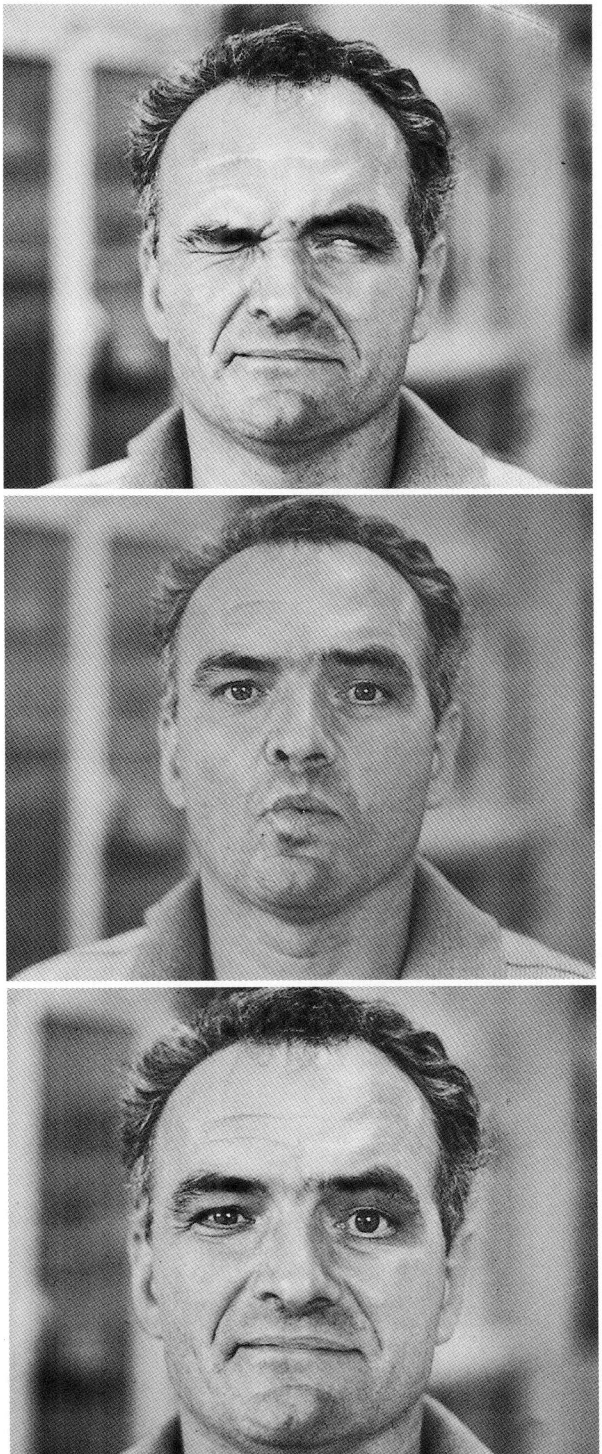

a

b

c

Fig. 1a–c. Facial nerve neuroma that developed in the mastoid portion of the fallopian canal with a preoperative facial paresis. A cable graft with the great auricular nerve was glued to the nerve endings with Tissucol. Grade IV recovery was noticed after 1 year. (From [3])

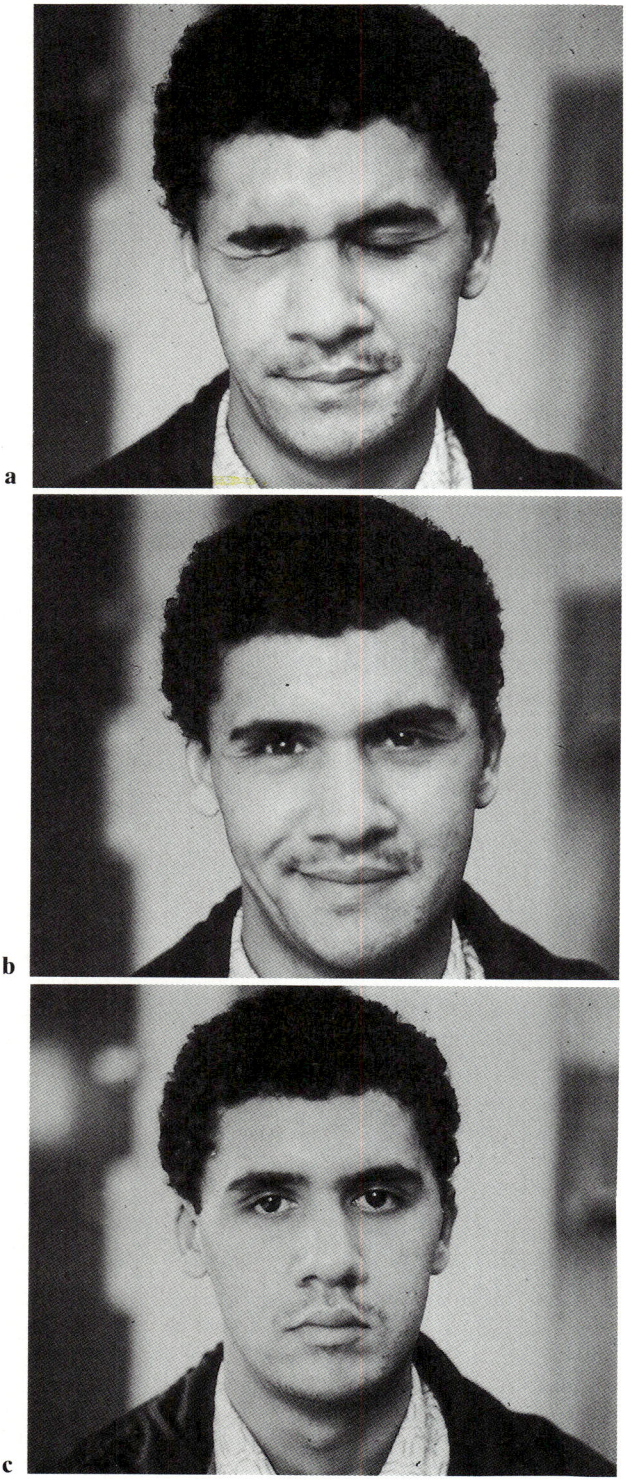

Fig. 2a–c. Iatrogenic section of the extracranial facial trunk into the parotid gland. Total repair of the facial nerve trunk and branches from the intratemporal mastoid portion of the nerve to the different branches of the nerve with two cable grafts using the sural nerve. Grade III recovery after 1 year. (From [3])

Table 3. Facial nerve function as a function of the pathology, localization, and the grafting technique one year after the anastomosis

	Grade III	IV	V	VI
CPA and IAC				
Termino-terminal	10	2	2	1
Cable graft	6	3	2	1
Hypoglosso-facial	4	4	–	–
Petrous bone and parotid gland				
Termino-terminal	1	–	1	–
Cable graft	10	5	–	–
Hypoglosso-facial	1	1	–	–

CPA, cerebellopontine angle; IAC, internal auditory canal.
The evaluation was done in 17 of 22 termino-terminal anastomoses, 27 of 32 cable graft anastomoses and 10 of 14 hypoglosso-facial anastomoses.

Results

The results were evaluated by two criteria: (1) observation of the first symptoms of regeneration before or after 6 months, (2) the House and Brackmann evaluation at 1 year. As shown in Table 3, the first signs of regeneration were observed before 6 months in two thirds of the patients when only one anastomosis has to be crossed (termino-terminal anastomosis or hypoglosso-facial anastomosis). Early regeneration was noticed in only 40 % of the cable graft anastomosis patients before 6 months. After 1 year, a good result (grades III and IV) was observed in 77 %, 89 %, and 100 % of the termino-terminal, cable graft, and hypoglosso-facial anastomosis, respectively. However, the best results (grade III) were observed for the termino-terminal anastomoses (65 %). For the cable graft and hypoglosso-facial anastomoses, grade III scores were obtained in 59 % and 50 % of the patients, respectively. No recovery of facial function (grade VI) was noticed in one patient with termino-terminal anastomosis (4 %) and one with cable graft anastomosis (5 %). A slight recovery (grade V) was observed in 18 % and 7 % of the termino-terminal and cable graft anastomosis patients, respectively. Lack of recovery (grades V and VI) was most often observed for grafts performed in the CPA or IAC (except for one patient with termino-terminal anastomosis in the petrous bone).

Discussion

Experimentally, fibrin glue anastomosis of the intratemporal facial nerve in the cat resulted in better recovery of facial function than an epineural suture or the natural union of the nerve endings [5]. Although no difference was observed clinically and histologically between the fibrin adhesive and the epineural suture, the magnitude of the summating potentials was higher after the former anastomosis than after the latter [5]. These observations demonstrate that fibrin adhesive is suitable for facial nerve anastomosis, with a limited perinervous fibrosis and nearly no foreign body reaction [2, 5, 6]. The best recovery that can be observed after a facial nerve grafting is a House and Brackmann's grade III and should be considered as a good recovery. This was best achieved when a termino-terminal anastomosis was performed. However, using a cable graft anastomosis, good and fair results were observed in nearly 90% of the patients.

Poor recovery was noticed for patients with termino-terminal anastomosis in the CPA for acoustic tumors and meningiomas. In the angle, the facial nerve has no perineural sheet [3, 7, 8], and is usually elongated and stretched by the tumor. A cable graft should be interposed between the nerve endings if the latter cannot be easily brought together. A rerouting of the intratemporal nerve may injure its vascularization and precludes good reinnervation. As demonstrated histologically by [5], fibrin adhesive does not penetrate between the nerve endings if they are well brought together without any traction and thus does not obstruct growth of the axons. Therefore the anastomosis should not be covered by any support or conjunctive sheet, as proposed by others [8].

References

1. Portmann M, Bébéar JP, Bagot-d'Arc M (1982) La colle de Fibrine (Tissucol) en otologie et neurotologie. A propos de nos 100 premiers cas. Rev Laryngol 103: 15–18
2. Siedentop KH, Loewy A (1979) Facial nerve repair with tissue adhesive. Arch Otolaryngol 105: 423–426
3. Sterkers O, Becherel P, Sterkers JM (1989) Réparation du nerf facial par colle de fibrine exclusive: 56 cas. Ann Oto-Laryngol 106: 176–181
4. House JW, Brackmann DE (1985) Facial nerve gradings system. Otolaryngol Head Neck Surg 93: 164–150
5. Bento RF, Minti A (1987) Comparison between fibrin tissue adhesive, epineural suture and natural union in intratemporal facial nerve of cats. Acta Otolaryngol Suppl (Stockh) 465: 1–36
6. Feldman MD, Sataloff RT, Epstein G, Ballas SK (1987) Autologous fibrin tissue adhesive for peripheral nerve anastomosis. Arch Otolaryngol 113: 963–967
7. Barrs MD, Brackmann DE, Hittelberger WE (1984) Facial nerve anastomosis in the cerebellopontine angle: a review of 24 cases. Am J Otol 5: 269–272
8. Fisch U, Dobic RA, Gunir A, Felix H (1987) Intracranial facial nerve anastomosis. Am J Otol 8: 23–29

III. Burns

Use of Human Fibrin Glue in Burn Wound Surgery

G. ARTURSON, A. HEDLUND, and S. VEDUNG

Abstract

Human fibrin glue has been used extensively to anchor skin, bone, and cartilage grafts to the recipient [1–3]. In patients with thermal injury there are some situations in which the combined benefits of fibrin glue for hemostasis and the stable fixation of the skin grafts to the wound surface might be of value. Literature findings and own experiences using human fibrin glue (Tisseel, Immuno AG, Vienna) in 25 patients (15–70 years old; 10%–60% body surface burn) indicate that this kind of procedure is of great value for fixation of skin grafts. The patients were also examined with respect to bacterial contamination of the wounds, neutrophil granulocyte functions and nutritional status, which is taken into account in the evaluation of the wound healing rate.

Introduction

Human fibrin glue has been used quite extensively to anchor skin, bone and cartilage grafts to the recipient [1–3]. In patients with thermal injury there are some situations in which the combined benefits of fibrin glue, hemostasis and stable fixation of the skin grafts to the wound surface, might be of value. The aim of the present investigation was to use human fibrin glue (Tisseel, Immuno AG, Vienna) for stable fixation of skin grafts following excision of particular types of deep burns in order to avoid formation of dead space and loosening or dislocation of the graft.

Materials and Methods

A total of 55 patients were studied, 34 men and 21 women. The age range was 15–70 years and the initial extent of the full-thickness burn was between 12% and 60% of the body surface area (BSA). In 32 patients 26 burns of the dorsum of the hands were excised within the first 2 days after injury. The skin grafts were then fixed with Tisseel. In 23 patients skin grafts were fixed with Tisseel on 29 granulating wounds with the following location: shoulders and axillas ($n = 9$); sides of the trunk ($n = 11$); gluteal folds ($n = 4$); and perineum

($n = 5$). Previous skin grafts to these 29 wounds failed to take. They occupied 0.5 %–3 % of BSA. All granulating wounds were cultured and the number of bacteria for each species was calculated. Antibiotics were given intravenously according to the results from the sensitivity tests. No topical antibiotics were used.

Burns larger than 20 % of BSA were all treated initially with parenteral fluids and nutrition, supplementary electrolytes, vitamins and trace elements. Excision and autografting of subdermal burns were performed when the patients had stabilized following resuscitation. In deep dermal and subdermal burns larger than 15 % of BSA we performed tangential excision and skin grafting in two or more procedures.

The skin grafts were fixed in place with Tisseel, applied using a spraying device. Standard nonadherent dressings were used.

Results

No general or local adverse effects were observed. When compared with the other methods used for securing skin grafts, fibrin glue was the only way to achieve adhesion of the whole surface. Fibrin glue added to the interface between the graft and the wound, occluded the dead space and safely anchored the grafts. We noticed no accumulation of blood or fluids underneath the skin grafts and no graft dislocation, although the patients ambulated to some extent after 2 days.

All patients with hand burns treated with immediate excision and fixation of the grafts with fibrin glue showed complete healing within 4 weeks, with excellent function of the hands. The time needed for the operation was reduced by about 50 % compared to the previous procedure when the grafts were fixed with sutures and strips.

All granulating wounds were contaminated. Bacteria such as *Staphylococcus albus* or *S. aureus, E. coli, Pseudomonas aeruginosa* or *Klebsiella* were cultured ($10–50^4$/gram tissue) from these wounds. Yet, they looked clean after revision at the time of skin grafting.

Of the 29 areas, 28 healed in 22 patients. An almost complete take of the skin grafts was obtained. The small residual defects healed spontaneously within 10 days. In only one patient, with a perineal wound and diarrhea, bowels infected the grafts, but the wound healed after an additional skin transplantation. There was stable and safe adhesion and little inflammatory reaction between the graft and the recipient area, resulting in favorable conditions for graft incorporation. By using the glue the last wounds in our patients healed earlier and the patients' general condition improved.

Discussion

As a first step in the adhesion of a skin graft to the wound surface a fibrin bridge is formed, following after a few days by the ingrowth of fibroblasts, fibrocytes and endothelium to incorporate the graft in the host. To develop the permanent collagen/elastin base between the graft and the wound the tissues must be sufficiently immobile in relation to one another, at least for a few days. Previous skin grafts in our patients failed because of motion of the grafts, sometimes caused by bleeding or infection. After firm fixation of the skin grafts to the host tissues by fibrin glue, we noticed neither dislocation nor formation of hematoma. Only one graft failure occurred, in a patient with a perineal wound and diarrhea.

Braun and coworkers [4] and Staindl [5] have shown that fibrin adhesive does not constitute a barrier to vascularization when used for fixation of skin grafts. The fibrin structure of the glue seems to serve as a matrix for ingrowing fibroblasts, and biopsies from skin grafts in burns have shown faster ingrowth of granulation tissue and fibroblasts after glueing [6]. Experimental use of the glue by Ohlsén et al. [2] also showed that the fibrin network is unbroken during the first week, but after that time degradation is rapid. After 2 weeks only a small amount of fibrin remains. Our patients were allowed some ambulation after a couple of days, but no dislocation of the skin was seen. Obviously, the fibrin glue is durable and strong enough to keep the transplant well fixed until sufficient healing has occurred.

Bösch [7] showed that bacterial growth is slower in a fibrin clot than in a physiological blood clot. The effect of fibrin glue on the healing of skin grafts in infected sites has also been tested by Jabs and coworkers [1]. When fibrin glue was added graft take was nearly the same in the infected and the noninfected wounds. In our patients no inflammatory reaction was noted in the transplanted area during the first week.

From these findings it might be assumed that fibrin stimulates the immune system to destroy the bacteria present. The fibrin added to the wound also may act by exceeding the bacterial enzymes' ability to digest fibrin.

The fibrinogen is manufactured' from pooled human plasma and, therefore, there is a potential danger of transmission of viral diseases, but no such complication has been reported. Autologous tissue glue made from the patient's own blood has been used [8], but it is difficult to get a sufficiently high concentration of fibrinogen and adhesive strength as in the homologous commercial product [9].

The most frequent cause of death after thermal injury is sepsis due to an impaired host defense reaction. Neutrophil granulocytes play a significant role in the resistance against infection, but in burn patients they often show an inhibition of chemotaxis and defects in phagocytosis indicating decreased capacity to combat invading bacteria [10, 11]. Therefore, in burn patients it is very important to cover the wounds as early as possible so that losses of water, electrolytes and proteins and the invasion of microbes are minimized. By using the glue the last wounds in our patients healed earlier and we believe they recovered sooner. Although no controlled randomized studies have been performed we consider the result as an improvement in the healing rate of these residual wounds, since the take of previous skin grafts had been very poor.

Conclusion

Literature findings and our own experience using human fibrin glue (Tisseel) in patients with burns indicate that this kind of procedure is of great value for fixation of skin grafts under the following circumstances:

1. In wound areas which are difficult to immobilize such as the neck, the axillas, perineum and the gluteal folds and sides of the trunk.
2. In slightly infected wounds after failure of previous ordinary skin graftings.
3. In some patients with poor nutritional status, e.g., with a defective immune response.
4. When careful hemostasis is important, mainly to avoid slow oozing from the wound surface.

References

1. Jabs AD, Wider T, DeBellis J, Hugo NE (1990) The effect of fibrin glue on skin grafts in infected sites. 59th Annual Meeting of the American Society of Plastic and Reconstructive Surgeons, 21–25 Oct 1990
2. Ohlsén L, Widenfalk B (1983) The early development of articular cartilage after perichondrial grafting. Scan J Plast Reconstr Surg 17: 163–177
3. Widenfalk B, Engkvist O, Ohlsén L, Segerström K (1986) Perichondrial arthroplasty using fibrin glue and early mobilization. Scan J Plast Reconstr Surg 20: 251–258
4. Braun F, Holle J, Kovac W, Lindner A, Spängler HP (1975) Untersuchungen über die Replantation autologer Vollhaut mit Hilfe von hochkonzentriertem Fibrinogen und Blutgerinnungsfaktor XIII. Wien Klin Wochenschr 14: 213–219
5. Staindl O (1977) Die Gewebeklebung mit hochkonzentriertem humanem Fibrinogen am Beispiel der freien, autologen Hauttransplantation. Arch Oto-Rhino-Laryngol 217: 219–228
6. Fisseler-Eckhoff A, Grabosch A, Donati I, Müller K-M (1988) Histologische Untersuchungen nach Hauttransplantation mit und ohne Fibrinkleber. Ellipse 15: 180–186
7. Bösch P (1981) Die Fibrinspongiosaplastik. Experimentelle Untersuchungen und klinische Erfahrungen. Wien Klin Wochenschr 124: 1–26
8. Siedentop K, Harris DM, Ham K, Sanches B (1986) Extended experimental and preliminary surgical findings with autologous fibrin tissue adhesive made from patient's own blood. Laryngoscope 96: 1062–1064
9. Laitakari K, Luotonen J (1989) Autologous and homologous fibrinogen sealants: adhesive strength. Laryngoscope 99: 974–976
10. Ransjö U, Forsgren A, Arturson G (1977) Neutrophil leucocyte functions and wound bacteria in burn patients. Burns 3: 171–173
11. Venge P, Arturson G (1981) Locomotion of neutrophil granulocytes from patients with thermal injury. Identification of serum derived inhibitors. Burns 8: 6–18

Tissucol: A 7-Year Experience in Burn Patients

Ch. Dhennin, L. Vesin, J. F. Feauveaux, J.-P. Berdalle,
and A. Yassine

Introduction

After third degree burn injuries, grafting remains the only way of healing. Delayed covering increases morbidity and mortality, whereas a high percentage of graft take guarantees wound closure and allows better long-term results.

To enable the skin grafts to take, they must be secured on their wound beds. Ideally, tie-over dressings provide the optimal result; unfortunately, they are most often useless for burn patients. In such cases, sutures, staples, strips, and fibrin glue [1–7] can be used; in some cases nothing is applied. In our burn center we have used Tissucol for 7 years. A review of our experience is presented here.

Preparation and Application of Tissucol

Preparation of the Tissucol components is best achieved with the equipment provided by Immuno, following the instructions. The preparation of Tissucol is very simple; reconstitution is completed after 10 min of heating in the Fibrinotherm with the human thrombin setting. However, some details are worth noting even if they appear minor: preheating the components for 5 min in the Fibrinotherm ensures optimum reconstitution, the entire lyophilized substance must be moistened, the right thrombin setting must obviously be chosen. Also foaming and clot formation is damaging; thus it is advisable to operate the magnetic stirrer and avoid manual methods. Similarly, only Fibrinotherm provides a precise and constant temperature of 37 °C.

During skin grafting, simultaneous spray application of the two reconstituted components appears to be the quickest and most reliable method. The necessary equipment consists of the filled syringes, Duploject, Spray-set and Tissomat (Immuno AG, Vienna).

Careful attention is required. It is particularly important to avoid foaming when drawing the constituents into the syringes; otherwise there is loss of expensive material and defective polymerization.

Tissucol is sprayed on the recipient bed [8] as a thin layer which can be seen as a translucent white deposit. Between 200 and 400 cm^2 are treated at each spraying. The grafts are spread immediately, ensuring that they do not wrinkle thereby sticking to themselves. The recipient bed must be prepared carefully. Sealing the grafts allows better adhesion but does not transform the recipient bed. Also hemostasis must be completely achieved or else the fibrin will allow coagulation but not sealing to take place. Our experience does not confirm other results [2].

Clinical Review

We reviewed the surgical records from January 1, 1985 to December 31, 1991. In this retrospective survey, only acute burn patients were studied. Amongst the patients hospitalized and receiving grafts, 315 benefited from the application of Tissucol. They sustained 510 surgical procedures for grafting at the time of early excision or later. The ages ranged from 14.5 to 91 years (mean = 43.5 ± 19.6 years). The total burn surface covered 1 % to 87 % (mean = 21.4 % ± 19.5 %) and the UBS index ranged from 2 to 337 (mean 60.2 ± 62.6).

The recipient bed was prepared by either excision to the fascia, tangential excision or scraping of the granulation tissue. The split-skin grafts, taken by a Brown dermatome, were meshed in ratios ranging from 1.5 to 9, according to the patient's needs. In some cases allografts were used. The areas covered during the operative procedures ranged from 50 to 6000 cm^2, with an average of 1320 ± 1000 cm^2.

No adverse effects were observed either locally or generally. Some problems did occur at the beginning but were quickly resolved by referring to the protocol. Sealing was achieved after 2–5 min except when there was bleeding. Neither wrinkling nor slipping were observed except on very small areas, despite some agitation in several patients. The results were similar regardless the recipient bed.

Discussion

The major advantages are safety, security, rapidity and simplicity:

1. *Safety* because of the bacteriological and biochemical controls, donor selection and viral inactivation by heating. In our experience we have never found any disease related to the product.
2. *Security* because the whole surface of the graft is sealed. Fibrin glue is the only method which allows this.
3. *Rapidity* because the application is completed in only a few minutes, as the glue is prepared at the same time as the recipient bed. This advantage is even more important when the area to be covered is larger, because it is dramatically important to reduce the operative and anesthetic time when large burns are concerned, especially on the core temperature level.
   Spraying is not painful, unlike sutures or staples, and there is no need to increase anesthesia at the end of the surgical procedure. As regards Tissucol itself, the introduction of human thrombin and the new methodology have

dramatically decreased the preparation time and increased the sealing power. However, the speed of polymerization has also increased, so that smaller areas must be covered in each spraying procedure because the time allowed for spreading the grafts on the recipient bed is shortened. Before human thrombin was introduced we used either the slow setting (thrombin 4) or the rapid setting diluted in a proportion 1 to 2. We have not yet experienced such a dilution with human thrombin.

4. *Simplicity* because of easier peri- and postoperative care. Nothing has to be removed, no time is wasted, and no pain occurs.

The one drawback of Tissucol is the cost, which is quite high. In France, the price is between 80 and 100 US dollars per milliliter. However, treatment of the burn patients is expensive and every additional cost must be compared with the advantages.

Conclusion

Obviously the results obtained with Tissucol justify a prospective and comparative study. Indeed the rate of graft take would be taken into account but its high success rate makes it difficult to compare it with and without Tissucol. Due to the possible role of the substance in wound repair, the healing time of meshed grafts [9], and long-term quality of the grafts could be investigated. Currently the enhancement of wound healing remains controversial [7] on the clinical and histological levels [10, 11] as does Tissucol's cost effectiveness.

References

1. Blümel G, Ascherl R, Haas S et al. (1986) Fibrin sealant in burn injuries – experimental study. Plastic Surgery Maxillofac Dent Surg 4: 98–103
2. Ihara N., Suzuki K, Tanaka H et al. (1984) Application of fibrin glue to burns. Its haemostatic and skin transplant fixation effects in the excised wound. Burns 10: 396–404
3. Pless J (1983) Fixation of skin grafts with Tisseel. In: Skjoldborg H (ed) Scientific Workshop 82. Tisseel/Tissucol-Symposium, pp 119–121
4. Saltz R, Dimick A, Harris C et al. (1989) Application of autologous fibrin glue in burn wounds. J Burn Care Rehabil 10: 504–507
5. Saltz R, Sierra D, Feldman D et al. (1991) Experimental and clinical applications of fibrin glue. Plast Reconstr Surg 6: 1005–1015
6. Saltz R (1992) Fibrin glue. Plast Reconstr Surg 90: 726–727
7. Staindl O (1983) Fibrin sealant in plastic surgery of head and neck. In: Skjoldborg H (ed) Scientific Workshop 82. Tisseel/Tissucol-Symposium, pp 97–104
8. Neuman AR, Weinberg A, Benmeir P et al. (1991) Spay application of fibrin glue by a simple device. Plast Reconstr Surg 88: 922–923
9. Boeckx W, Vandevoort M, Blondeel P et al. (1992) Fibrin glue in the treatment of dorsal hand burns. Burns 18:395–400
10. Harmand MF, Michel D, Bagot d'Arc M et al. (1986) Effect of fibrin seals on human fibroblast attachment and multiplication. European Congress on Biomaterials, 1986, Bologna
11. Piechotta FU, Flemming I (1983) The maximization of wound healing with fibrin glue. Aesthet Plast Surg 7: 81–82

The Use of Fibrin Sealant in Burn Treatment

D. L. Dyess, C. Blache, T. Wright, J. R. Fletcher, and A. Luterman

Abstract

Tangential excision is currently recommended for the care of deep dermal and full thickness burn injuries. A major problem in the technique is the blood loss that occurs with the excision. This blood loss has been one of the major deterrents to the ubiquitous acceptance of this technique. Tangential excision shortens hospital stay. The general opinion among burn surgeons is that cosmesis and function are also substantially improved.

A new technique using fibrin sealant (Tisseel, Immuno) has been tested at our institution as part of a multi-institutional trial in the United States. Burn wounds are excised with a tourniquet in place after the arm is milked of blood using an Esmark Bandage. Fibrin sealant is then applied using a spraying device. Split-thickness skin grafts are applied and a second layer of sealant is sprayed over the grafts to secure them. The tourniquet is then released. Standard, nonadherent dressings are used.

Sixteen patients were entered into the clinical study at the University of South Alabama Burn Center. The average age of the patients was 34.3 ± 5.2 years, and the average percent total body surface area burned was 24.9 ± 5.5 TBSA. There were 13 males and three females. The average area excised was 149.7 ± 26.6 square inches. There was excellent take of the grafts with rapid closure of the interstices [graft take (% ± SE) = 87.6% ± 4.38%, median = 95%], [time to interstices closure (% ± SE) = 5.6 ± .5 days, median = 6 days]. There was no slippage of the skin grafts despite the lack of use of staples or sutures. The grafts were secured soley with the fibrin sealant. Blood loss at the excision and graft site was reduced to minimal amounts (10 cc).

In summary, fibrin sealant is a dramatic and exciting new adjunct currently under evaluation in the United States for tangential excision and split-thickness skin grafts. Further studies are being developed to document efficacy and cost effectiveness.

Introduction

A major problem encountered in managing burn victims is blood loss from tangential excision of the burn wound. This often limits the extent of debridement or excision that can be performed at an operative procedure. Following excision, coverage of the burn wound requires securing split-thickness skin grafts to the excised wound. Present methods of securing these grafts have certain disadvantages: suturing techniques greatly extend operative time, staples are painful and time-consuming to remove, and adhesive tapes do not secure the grafts well.

In 1909, Bergel [1] documented the hemostatic effectiveness of fibrin powder. This important finding was the beginning of a new era in the field of surgical adhesives. Reports soon followed of the success of fibrin sealant as an adhesive in many types of surgery. Grey [2] reported the efficacy of fibrin for hemostasis in cerebral surgery. The first reports of fibrin as a means for fixation of skin grafts were in 1944 by Cronkite [3] and Tidrick [4].

Fibrin sealant, commercially available as Tisseel (Immuno AG, Vienna, Austria), has been widely used by European surgeons since the 1970s. This product is a two-component fibrin sealant prepared from fibrinogen (made from pooled human plasma) and thrombin.

Fibrin sealant has been proposed as beneficial in the operative management of burn victims. Suggested indications for its use include:

1. Hemostasis
2. Securing autografts
3. Sealing donor sites

Fibrin sealant was evaluated at the University of South Alabama as part of a multi-institutional trial to determine the efficacy of Tisseel in the operative management of burn victims. This study adhered to the Human Review Guidelines of the University of South Alabama Investigational Review Board, which approved the protocol. The following report summarizes the experience at the University of South Alabama Burn Center.

Materials and Methods

Patient Population

Adult patients admitted to the University of South Alabama Burn Center were considered for this study. Only those requiring operative intervention for management of burn wounds greater than 10% total body surface area were eligible. Following informed consent, patients were entered into the study. Patients were managed by established treatment regimens for all aspects of their injury, with the exception of the use of fibrin sealant at the time of surgical intervention.

Preparation of Fibrin Sealant

The fibrin sealant used in this study was Tisseel. This product was provided in a kit containing the following four components: freeze-dried sealer protein concentrate; freeze-dried thrombin (500 units); calcium chloride (40 m*M* in

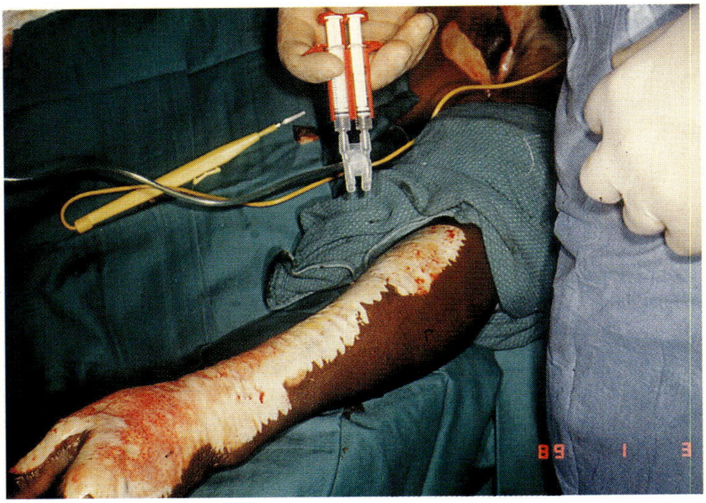

Fig. 1. Tisseel being applied to excised arm

1 ml volume); and fibrinolysis inhibitor (aprotinin solution 3000 KIU in 1 ml volume). The protein concentrate was dissolved in the solution of fibrinolysis inhibitor, hereafter referred to as the sealant solution. The thrombin was reconstituted in the calcium chloride solution, referred to as the thrombin solution. Each of these solutions was prepared and then agitated on a fibrinotherm, a combined heating and stirring device, to simplify reconstitution of the highly concentrated sealer proteins.

Application of Fibrin Sealant

The fibrin sealant was applied by a spray system consisting of a Duploject applicator, a spray head, and a pressure controlling device (Tissomat). The Duploject sterile applicator system consisted of a syringe holder and common plunger for two identical disposable syringes, a needle holder and an application needle. Using this system, the two-component solutions were injected separately into a continuous gas jet. As the droplets bombarded each other in the air and on the wound surface, mixing occurred to form a fibrin film (Fig. 1).

Surgical Techniques

Fibrin sealant was applied during the surgical procedures for the following indications: (1) hemostasis; (2) securing autograft, or (3) donor site sealing. The sealant was applied to a total body surface area of 3 %–5 % in each patient when used for hemostasis or securing autograft. Povidone iodine was not used for either prepping or for dressings as this compound interferes with the con-

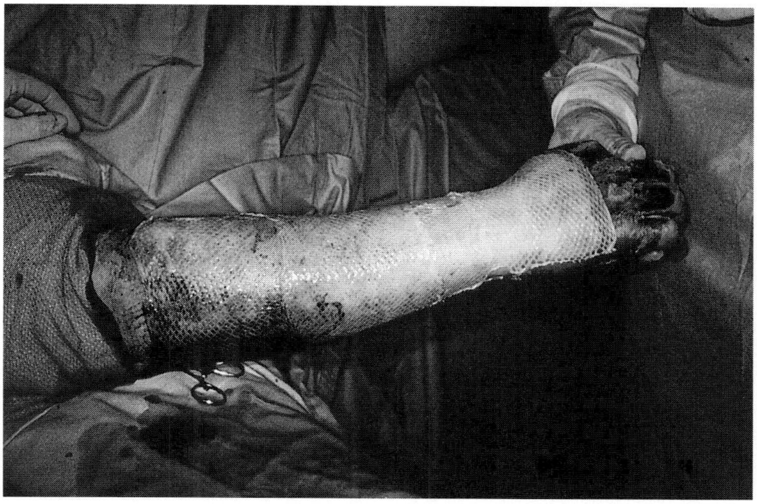

Fig. 2. Tourniquet released, minimal blood loss

version of fibrinogen to fibrin. The following specific techniques were used for application of the agent.

Hemostasis. The injured area to be excised for each patient was randomly divided into two equal areas, the control site and the test area, with each site representing at least 5 % of the total body surface area. Immediately following tangential excision of the burn wound, fibrin sealant (Tisseel) was applied to the test site wound bed and allowed to "set" for 5 min. Meshed split-thickness autografts (0.012–0.016 inches thick) were placed and secured with staples, then the wounds were dressed with saline-saturated outer dressings. The outer dressing is a commercially available product that consists of three layers. The inner layer is a nonadherent wound contact layer, the middle layer an absorbent cotton layer, and the outer layer is a nonocclusive layer. These layers are bound together at the edges to produce one dressing. The control site was immediately treated according to the standard technique of the University of South Alabama Burn Center. This included application of topical thrombin to the wound bed, then covering the bed with Telfa saturated with epinephrine/saline. Hot laparotomy sponges were placed on top of the Telfas, then the extremity was wrapped with an Ace elastic wrap. This was allowed to remain in place approximately 10 min. After removal, a split-thickness skin graft was applied and secured with staples, then dressed with a saline-saturated Exudry dressing.

Securing Autograft. A sterile tourniquet was positioned proximally on the burned extremity. An Esmark's bandage was used to wrap the extremity, "milking" the blood from the limb. The tourniquet was then inflated to 1.5 times systolic blood pressure and the Esmark's bandage was removed. The burn wound was tangentially excised, then fibrin sealant was applied and allowed to dry for 5 min. Meshed split-thickness skin grafts (0.012–0.016 inches thick) were positioned on the wound bed, then fibrin sealant was applied to the surface of the grafts. Another 5 min drying period followed, then the tourniquet was released and the wounds dressed (Fig. 2).

Donor Site Sealing

Each patient's donor site was randomly divided into two equal areas, the control site and the test area. A dermatome was used to harvest skin 10–12 thousandths of an inch thick.

The control site was immediately treated according to the standard technique of the University of South Alabama Burn Center. This included application of topical thrombin to the wound bed, then covering the bed with Telfa saturated with epinephrine/saline. Hot laparotomy sponges were placed on top of the Telfas, then the extremity wrapped with an Ace elastic wrap. This was allowed to remain in place approximately 10 min. After removal, the wound bed was dressed with an occlusive dressing.

Immediately after the graft was harvested from the test area, fibrin sealant was applied to the donor wound site and allowed to dry for 5 min. The donor site was then dressed with an occlusive dressing (Opsite).

Clinical Observations

Blood loss was evaluated for each operative procedure by preoperative weighing of all sponges, gauzes and drapes used for the procedure, and then again weighing these postoperatively.

Graft Take

Dressings for skin grafts were allowed to remain undisturbed for 3 days, unless wound cultures obtained at the time of surgery indicated the growth of bacteria or the patient became febrile. Dressings were removed prior to 3 days at the occurrence of either of these events. Dressings were removed by a nurse clinical specialist (blinded observer), leaving the inner layer of the outer dressing in situ. The sites were examined twice daily after the initial dressings were removed. Assessment included the following: (1) percentage take; (2) infection; and (3) speed of closure of interstices of mesh graft. Cultures were taken prior to the onset of antibacterial treatment if purulence developed. Photographs were taken on every other day for 2 weeks.

Patient Preference

Patients were interviewed by a blinded observer. The patients were asked to compare the test areas (sites where fibrin sealant was applied) to the control areas for severity of pain and pruritus. Linear analogue visual scales (range 1–10) were used for this assessment.

Speed of Epithelialization and Pigmentation

The speed at which epithelial coverage was achieved was determined by a blinded observer. Photographs were taken at weekly intervals of the test area and control site. Any specific problems such as cellulitis were recorded. Infections were treated in accordance with standard methods of care for the University of South Alabama Burn Center.

Patient Follow-up

A blinded observer examined the control site and the test area at monthly intervals in the outpatient clinic for a period of 6 months. The wounds were evaluated for speed of repigmentation, presence or absence of hypertrophic scarring and persistence of pruritus. Patients were also interviewed for their preference (Figs. 3, 4).

Results

A total of 16 patients were entered into the clinical study at the University of South Alabama, 13 males and three females. The age range of the group was 5–80 years, with an average age of 34.3 ± 5.2 years. The average percent total body surface area burned was 24.9 % ± 5.5 %, with a range of 4 %–75 %. The

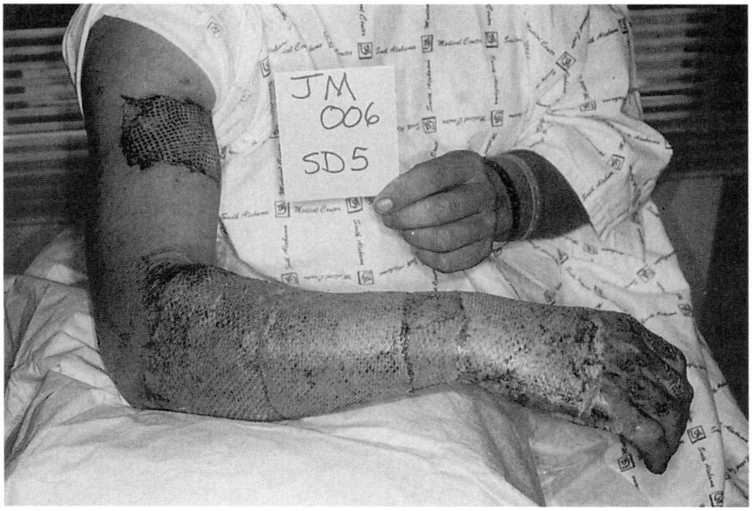

Fig. 3. Postoperative day 6: closure of interstices

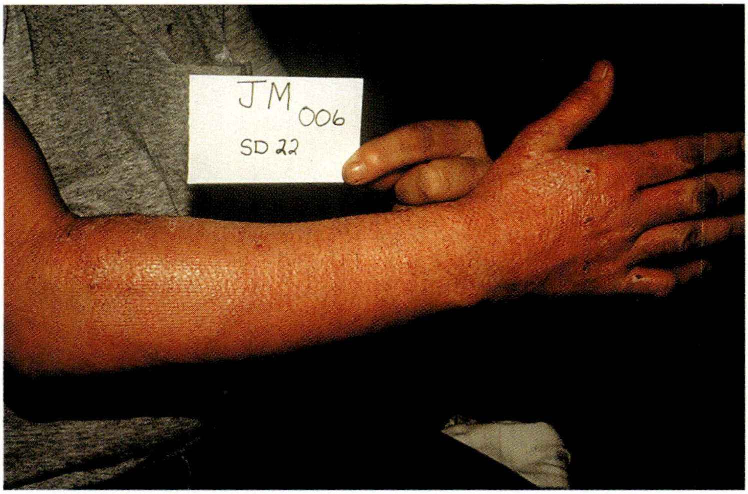

Fig. 4. Postoperative day 28: full function restored

average time from admission to the Burn Center until the surgical procedure utilizing fibrin sealant was 11 days, with a median time of 3.5 days. The procedure in which fibrin sealant was used was not always the initial operative intervention, explaining the mean of 11 days.

Fibrin sealant was used in eight patients predominantly for hemostasis following tangential excision, and in eight patients as a means of securing split-thickness skin graft and for hemostasis. The agent was used for sealing a donor site in only one patient. The average area excised was 966 ± 171.6 cm^2, with a range of 193.5–1935.5 cm^2.

Fibrin sealant was applied to burn wounds in the following locations: neck (three patients); upper extremities (eight patients); lower extremities (five patients); anterior trunk (one patient); posterior trunk (two patients). Tisseel was applied to more than one body location in three patients.

When fibrin sealant was used to provide hemostasis of the excised wound bed, the blood loss was minimal. The total blood loss for each burn wound was less than 10 ml when fibrin sealant was used for hemostasis on extremity wounds excised under tourniquet. The tourniquet inflation time was always less than 30 min.

There was excellent take of the grafts with rapid closure of the interstices. The average "take" for the grafts was 87.6% ± 4.38%. The time interval for closure of the interstices was 5.6 days (0.5 S.E., median 6 days). There was no slippage of the skin grafts despite the lack of use of staples or sutures. The grafts were secured using only fibrin sealant.

Discussion

The blood loss associated with excision of severe burn injury is often the limiting factor in the surgical management of these patients. Studies by Moran et al. [5] reported an average loss of 196 ml of blood for each percent of the body excised using the technique of tangential excision. Goodwin et al. [6] reported an average blood loss of 1270 ml from tangential excision of a single hand burn – approximately 2 % of the total body surface area of a patient. Rosenberg and Zawaki [7] reduced the mean blood loss to 29 ml per percent body surface area excised by the use of the tourniquets. The technique of fibrin sealant and tourniquet in combination is clearly significant in the reduction of blood loss associated with excision of the burn wound.

Warden et al. [8] described an alternative method of decreasing blood loss which involved returning the patient to the operating room 24 h following the initial excision for application of split-thickness skin grafts. The average blood loss reported for this technique was 0.72 ml/cm^2 excised when tourniquets were used, and 1.26 ml/cm^2 when tourniquets were not used [8]. Using the results of this study to predict blood loss, we would have expected the loss of greater than 800 ml blood per excision, as our average excised area was 950 cm^2. When the burns were excised under tourniquet and Tisseel applied, the average blood loss was less than 10 ml.

The next question we addressed was the effectiveness of Tisseel in securing grafts. In our patients, we had no slippage of grafts and rapid closure of the interstices. The rapid closure is most likely related to the closed system created by the sealant; however, it is possible that it has growth stimulating effects. This finding requires further study.

In conclusion, our results suggest that Tisseel is effective, with proven clinical benefit, both as a hemostatic agent and in securing grafts in the operative management of burn wounds.

References

1. Bergel S (1909) Über Wirkungen des Fibrins. Dtsch Med Wochenschr 35: 663
2. Grey EG (1915) Fibrin as a hemostatic in cerebral surgery. Surg Gynecol Obstet 21: 452
3. Cronkite EP, Lozner EL, Deaver J (1944) Use of thrombin and fibrinogen in skin grafting. JAMA 124: 976
4. Tidrick RT, Warner ED (1944) Fibrin fixation of skin transplants. Surgery 15: 90
5. Moran KT, O'Reilly TJ, Furman W et al. (1988) A new algorithm for calculation of blood loss in excisional burn surgery. Am Surg 54: 207–208
6. Goodwin CW, Maguire MS, McManus WF et al. (1983) Prospective study of burn wound excision of the hands. J Trauma 23: 510–517
7. Rosenberg JL, Zawacki BE (1986) Reducing of blood loss using tourniquets and "compression" dressings in excising limb burns. J Trauma 26: 47–50
8. Warden GD, Saffle JR, Kravitz M (1982) A two-stage technique for excision and grafting of burn wounds. J Trauma 22: 98–103

Skin Grafting with Fibrin Glue in Burns

J. P. Adant, B. Detroz, M. D'Silva, L. Natowitz, M. Ledoux,
B. Pestiaux, and P. Leclercq

Abstract

In an attempt to obtain better function and appearance, minimize blood loss and increase graft survival with minimal postoperative care, deep burns are treated by applying fibrin glue to difficult recipient sites.

We use a two-component fibrin sealant: fibrinogen made from pooled human plasma and bovine thrombin (Tissucol, Immuno AG, Vienna, Austria). The fibrin sealant is described as well as the technique used to seal the skin grafts in 15 patients (18 procedures). Graft sealing is limited to grafts located over areas subject to movement (joints, face, neck, hands) and to nonmeshed grafts for cosmetic reasons.

Our clinical experience, described here, demonstrates several advantages of sealing skin grafts on burn wounds: (1) hemostasis, early adherence and wound healing are improved; (2) better cosmetic results are obtained with sheet grafts on the face and neck; (3) operating time is reduced; (4) no special dressings are required; physiotherapy starts after 24 h; the recovery period is reduced as are secondary procedures.

Introduction

Early tangential excision and immediate grafting of the burn injured patient is the rule in burn centers. However, this technique involves the potential for significant blood loss, prolonged operative time, partial loss of graft due to underlying hematoma and to subsequent infection [1].

Very often, burn patients fail to meet the indications for receiving a graft for several reasons: (1) The area that has to be grafted shows necrosis resulting in poor chances of vascularization. (2) There is often a coagulopathy with resulting hematoma underneath the graft reducing the chances of success. (3) Nearly all the wounds are infected. (4) Due to the necessary intensive therapy of the severely burned patient, it is nearly impossible to immobilize the grafted areas.

The use of fibrin glue has already provided evidence for its positive hemostatic and skin transplant fixation effects [2–4]. We limited our study to certain indications: (1) Grafts over areas which are mechanically strongly affected by motion, e.g., face, joints, neck, and hands. (2) Grafts which are not meshed for cosmetic reasons (face, grafting in children).

The concept of fibrin fixation of skin grafts dates as far back as 1944 when Cronkite reported the use of topical thrombin and plasma for fixation of skin grafts [4, 5]. Since then, applications of fibrin glue have increased in many different surgical procedures including microvascular anastomoses, neurosurgery, plastic surgery and ear, nose and throat surgery [3, 6–9]. Recently, patients with burn wounds have been treated with human keratinocytes cultured on fibrin glue [19]

In our study we used a two-component preparation: fibrin, made from a human protein concentrate, and thrombin (Tissucol). When the two solutions are combined, thrombin, in the presence of calcium converts fibrinogen into fibrin. Factor XIII, a fibrin stabilizing factor present in blood, will convert fibrin monomer into fibrin polymer. Aprotinin, an antiplasmin substance is added to protect the fibrin polymer clot from premature fibrinolysis (Fig. 1), since in infected burn wounds, fibrinolytic activity is high [5, 6, 10, 11].

Fibrin glue works as an adhesive by emulating the exudative phase of wound healing. This may be specifically attributed to the presence of factor XIII, which is known to accelerate the exudative process. At the end of this phase there is formation of a stable fibrin structure that facilitates the growth of collagen producing fibroblasts. This stable fibrin matrix is fundamental to wound edge adhesion and wound healing [12–15].

Histological studies are not definitive but sealed grafts seem to show fewer inflammatory reactions (perivascular edema and bleeding, perivascular round cell infiltration) under the grafts than nonsealed ones. There is no irritating foreign body effect or granulation formation after incorporation because of the biological quality of the glue [10, 16].

Fibrin glue is obtained from pooled human plasma. The main danger of this pooled preparation is the transmission of viral diseases such as viral hepati-

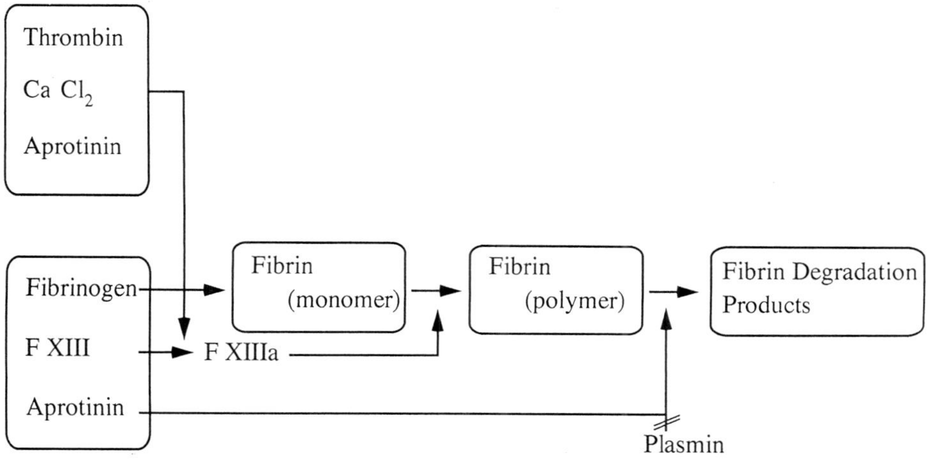

Fig. 1. Working principle of fibrin glue

tis and AIDS. Nevertheless, with careful donor selection and control and by the use of thermal viral inactivation it is possible to avert the transmission of such viruses. There has been no report of seroconversion after such a procedure [17, 18].

The following represents our experience in 15 patients, in whom fibrin glue was used on critical areas and/or for cosmetic reasons.

Materials and Methods

The 15 patients in whom fibrin glue was utilized are listed in Table 1. Indications for sealing were: grafts over stressed areas and cosmetic grafts. All of the patients sustained their injuries by flame, and 18 procedures were performed utilizing fibrin glue. This does not represent all procedures performed on this group of patients.

The extent of the burns varied from 5 % of total body surface area to 50 %, averaging 26.3 % (deep burns). There were eight women and seven men. The range was from 2 to 70 years, averaging 27.6 years.

Burns were first treated locally with Flammacerium (Duphar B.V. Amsterdam, The Netherlands). Most were treated with hydrotherapy, debridement and topical antibacterials. Infection is the rule in burn wounds. Examination of the areas we intended to graft showed contamination by *Staphylococcus aureus, Streptococcus faecalis, Pseudomonas aeruginosa, Candida albicans* and others. We carried out necrectomies after systemic stabilization and exact demarcation of the deep burned area (deep second degree or third degree burns).

As a rule, we fixed the grafts during the same operation or a few hours postoperatively in the intensive care unit. We sealed both mesh grafts and sheets.

Skin grafts were generally 3:1 meshed autografts. However, where noted, full-thickness or split-thickness *nonmeshed* grafts were also used when cosmetic result was important (children, face, neck).

Only one patient died in the burn unit during this evaluation period, from endobronchial burns. At that time graft take was 95 %. No seroconversion was noted in this group. Routine investigations showed no signs of hepatitis although acute transfusion of whole blood had to be administred in several patients.

More than 90 % of the area of the grafts we sealed by fibrin glue were accepted in most cases. Failures were due to infection and/or hematoma. In some cases, symmetrical areas were compared: one side with fibrin sealant and the other one without. Partial loss of graft was more frequent in nonsealed areas: 20 %–25 % compared to 5 %–10 % in sealed areas (Fig. 2).

Facial burns that had not healed at 10 days were tangentially excised down to the viable tissue and immediately grafted with medium-thickness skin sheet grafts. These were obtained from the most suitable donor site available with an appropriate match in color and in texture (scalp, supraclavicular areas) and respected facial aesthetic units [20].

The method was standardized. We used Tissucol lyophilized in combination with fibrinotherm S, which proved to be an excellent warming and stirring

Table 1. Characteristics of patients treated with fibrin glue

Patient	Age/sex	Body surface area (%)	Post-burn days	Grafted area	Graft take (%)	Comments
1	57/F	45	60	Buttocks	95	Excellent adherence; healing of 3:1 meshed grafts on an infected area
2	37/M	15	5	Popliteal fossa	100	Rapid healing; no limitation of knee motility
3	70/F	40	4	Right hand	95	Death from respiratory infection
4	4/F	30	5	Right leg	100	No blood loss (500 U thrombin)
5	30/F	25	5	Neck	100	Nonmeshed grafts; no hematoma (500 U thrombin)
6	28/F	35	44	Left axilla	100	Excellent adherence; open treatment
7	2/F	20	11	Chest, shoulder	100	Open treatment; no blood loss
8	10/M	15	10	Chest,	90	Meshed grafts; open treatment
				neck	100	Nonmeshed grafts; open treatment
			16	Scalp,	95	Meshed grafts
			16	shoulder	90	Meshed grafts
			20	Face	100	Nonmeshed grafts; open treatment (500 U thrombin)
9	12/M	10	10	Face	100	Nonmeshed grafts; open treatment
10	14/F	5	4	Neck	100	Nonmeshed grafts; no transfusion
11	50/M	10	6	Neck	100	Nonmeshed grafts; open treatment; no blood loss
12	22/M	45	10	Neck	100	Nonmeshed grafts; open treatment
			20	Shoulder	90	Meshed grafts; open treatment
13	30/F	40	20	Face, neck	95	Nonmeshed grafts; open treatment
14	12/M	10	5	Left ankle	100	Rapid healing; no limitation of ankle motility
15	37/M	50	20	Back	90	No blood loss; no hematoma (500 U thrombin)

device for the standardized reconstitution of fibrin sealant. The fibrin sealant solution and the thrombin solution are ejected from two separate jets under a pressure of 2 atm and blend as they are sprayed, in two overlapping cones, across the surface to be sealed (Duploject application system). By spraying at a distance of approximately 15 cm, the two components are evenly distributed across a circular area (1 ml over 100 cm^2) and result in a delicate fibrin film to avoid producing a further diffusion barrier under the graft.

After tangential excision of the burn injured tissues, identifiable bleeding sites were cauterized. This provided a bed that required additional hemostasis

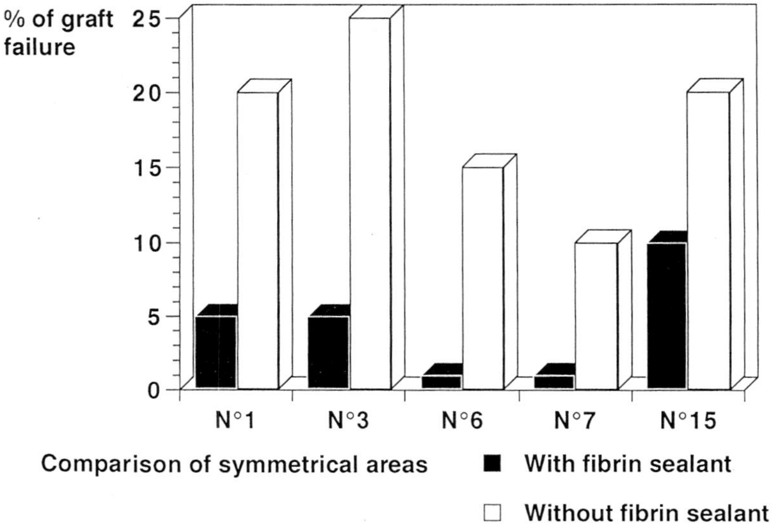

Fig. 2. Percent of graft failure in symmetrical areas: one side with fibrin sealant and the other without

secondary to multiple capillary bleeding. At this time the wound was dried with sponges, and fibrin glue was immediately sprayed [3, 9].

The concentration of thrombin (4 IU/ml or 500 IU/ml) determines the rapidity of reaction; with 500 IU/ml concentration, solidification of the formed clot is almost immediate (within 30 s of application). We used it for quick hemostasis and adhesion.

Special attention was given to the fact that unconsolidated fibrin sealant might be washed away by extravasation of blood from the surrounding tissue. Manipulations and shifting of tissues were avoided during these few minutes of consolidation of the fibrin sealant (with 4 IU/ml concentration), but gentle, uniform pressure was applied over the entire graft for 2 or 3 min immediately after the glue was applied.

As far as possible, dressings were avoided postoperatively. Further treatment was along similar lines. Hematomas and any fluid that had collected beneath the nonmeshed grafts were evacuated and the grafts were aspirated with an insulin syringe.

Early and easier mobilization was possible. There was no crusty adhesion of bandages causing pain and tearing the grafts when removed. The operative surface was dry and without pain. For 72 h the grafts were kept humid by spraying Ringer's solution over the grafted area.

Results

Adhesion Effects

One of the major problems in skin grafting is graft sliding by lack of adhesion, particularly on certain areas which are strongly stressed in motion, e.g., face, joints, neck, and axilla. In those cases, anchoring of the graft by stitches, acrylate glue (Histoacryl) or special dressings is rather difficult [2, 4, 5, 8, 16, 21].

The use of fibrin glue allows excellent and immediate biological adhesion with perfect application of the graft on the sealed area. It ensures intimate contact between the graft and the recipient site leading to higher rates of graft incorporation, as in nonmeshed grafts.

Further evidence of adhesion can be extrapolated by the overall take of grafts, which is more than 90%. These excellent results in graft take occur under a variety of conditions from meshed grafts at 3:1 expansion to full-thickness nonmeshed grafts and to open treatment of non-immobilized, non-stitched grafts on the face and neck.

Fibrin glue use avoids bolster-type dressings and long-term immobilization. This allows a full range of motion earlier in the postoperative period, reducing the rehabilitation period and limiting contractures. Some of the patients did not suffer any limitation of joint motion. Others needed secondary reconstructive procedures (flaps) to regain joint motion. Primary closure of the burn wound and thus protection against infection are the main goals. It appears that the use of fibrin glue reduces the number of secondary procedures. Also, with biological glue, there is no dead space and so the incidence of infection is reduced. Nevertheless, some of patients with good early results will also need reconstructive procedures because of scar contractures.

Hemostatic Effects

In many cases, hemorrhage caused by tangential excision is a crucial factor limiting the extent of such procedures. Due to the highly variable nature of the burn injury, estimation of blood loss in the immediate perioperative phase is often inaccurate. Nevertheless, we found the hemostatic value of fibrin glue in the tangentially excised wound to be clearly beneficial. Ihara et al. showed a 60% reduction in blood transfusion need in their group treated with fibrin glue [2].

The tissue surface should be as dry as possible immediately prior to application of the components to allow maximal adhesion of the fibrin glue. Clot formation occurs within seconds of application. Hemostasis and amount of blood loss are markedly improved by using fibrin glue, in particular with the 500 IU/ml thrombin concentration.

The fibrin sealant not only serves as a clotting agent but also minimizes hematoma formation both peri- and postoperatively. Patients with nonmeshed grafts benefit significantly from this technique. Moreover, preventing hematoma formation reduces the incidence of infection.

Healing

Marked improvement in hemostasis and graft adhesion are combined with an excellent rate of graft healing. Graft survival was more than 90%. The losses were generally due to failure to recognize fluid collection during the immediate postoperative period. There was no impaired healing [22].

A skin graft depends for its immediate viability upon nutrients from tissue fluids exuding from the recipient bed (plasmatic imbibition) [23]. Furthermore, fibrin sealing is an excellent aid to vascularization during the first few postoperative days and enhances rapid wound healing by primary intention. Fibrin glue provides a stable matrix for fibroblasts producing collagen. After 3 days, vascularization starts, which is decisive for further healing [23]. Especially within these first days, this tender vascularization can be disturbed. A profuse exudate typical of an infected wound or hematoma following insufficient hemostasis prevents contact between graft and wound.

Full-thickness grafts require a well vascularized bed but split-skin grafts can take well on a bed of doubtful vascularity which is frequently present. Full-thickness grafts are less likely to undergo subsequent contraction. Grafted areas also develop hypertrophy at the margins of the graft and sometimes in the graft bed itself, particularly when the grafts are thin [20].

In the postoperative period, we avoid the use of additional dressings. Changes, of wound dressings are highly painful, and often causes bleeding because of sheering, which may destroy the stitching of the grafts or disrupt the young vessels. Moreover, exposure to the air reduces the chance of *Pseudomonas* infection.

Discussion

In none of the patients did we encounter an adverse effect after the application of fibrin sealant. Fibrin sealing yields better appearance and function than that obtained by traditional treatments. Healing of grafts was rapid, allowing early mobilization of the joint and thus early rehabilitation. The great disadvantage of early surgical excision is that movement is not possible for a 5 day period after skin graft application and stiffness is therefore temporarily increased. The donor area may be likewise coated with fibrin sealant, so that the patient could be instantly mobilized and is able to leave his/her bed for physical therapy owing to a relative absence of pain. Patients are able to eat and move around on the first postoperative day without pressure dressings.

Skin meshing allows both expansion of the donor skin and drainage of the recipient bed. This technique is used where there is either a donor site shortage or suspected contamination of the recipient bed. The bare areas in the mesh are covered by epithelial migration from the grafted margins once the graft has taken.

With fibrin glue, nonmeshed grafts can be used more frequently, giving a better functional and aesthetic restoration. We also use thicker grafts (medium split- to full-thickness) which are durable, have a more natural texture and con-

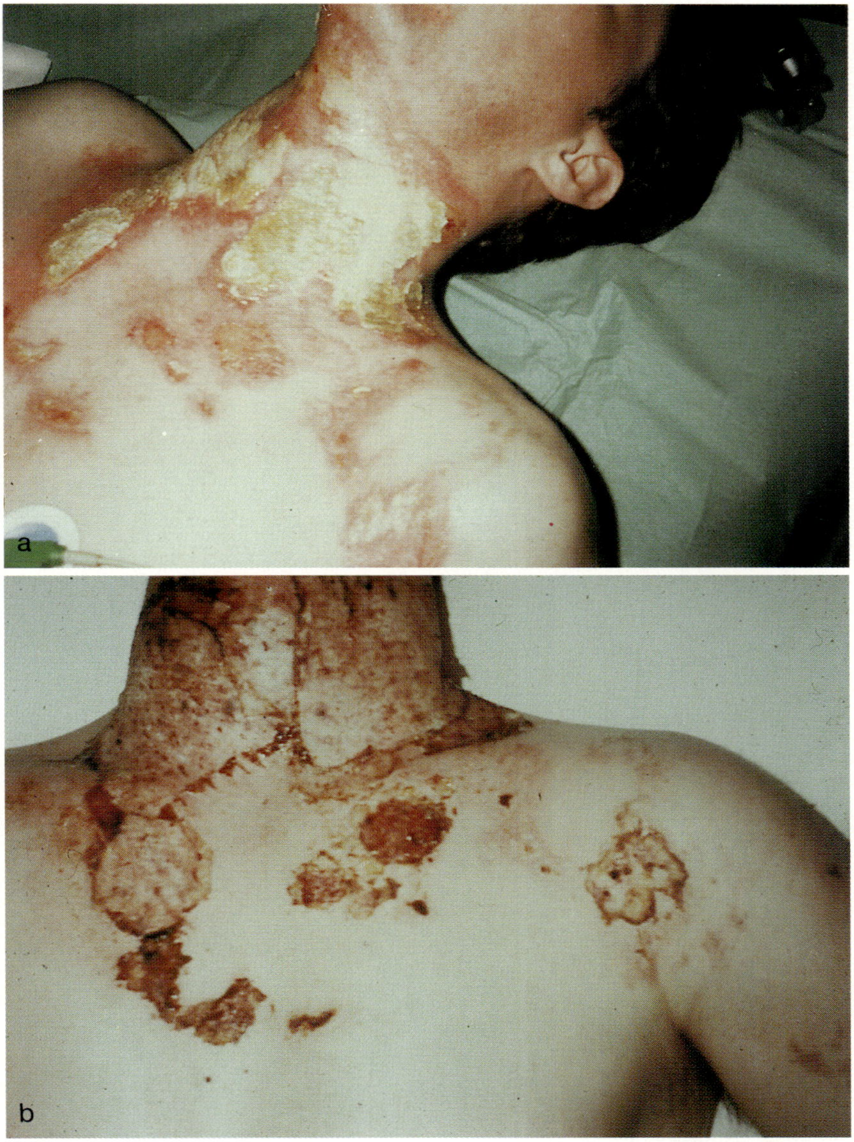

Fig. 3. **a** Deep burns on the neck; **b** Nonmeshed skin grafts on the same neck after excision. With fibrin glue, grafts are perfectly adherent

tract less. They have a certain inherent elasticity which allows them to stretch on movement. However, thicker grafts take less well on recently traumatized beds. The take of such grafts is proportional to their thickness during the phase of plasmatic imbibition. Reconstructive procedures, when required, were of lesser magnitude, especially with facial burns.

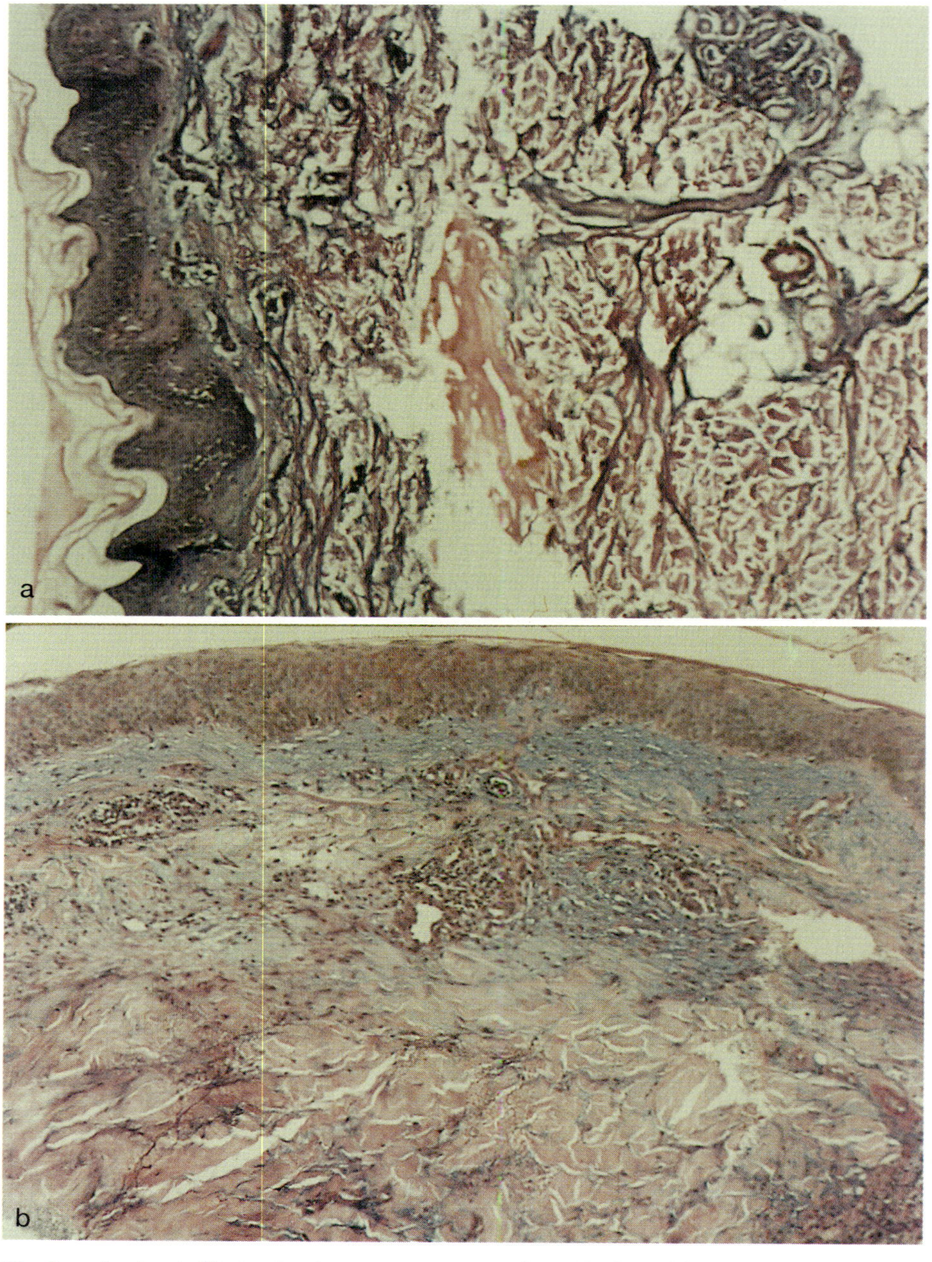

Fig. 4. **a** At day 1, fibrin glue is seen as an amorphous PAS-positive substance between the skin graft and the reticular dermis. **b** At day 5, fibrin glue is completely resorbed without scar formation

No apparent negative effect with regard to infection was observed. Infection is reduced for several reasons: no dead space, no hematoma and early excision of burn wounds. Certain authors [12, 24] suggest that fibronectin, present in fibrin glue, gives an antiseptic effect. Fibronectin stimulates bacterial phagocytosis and so reduces infection [24].

When symmetrical areas were compared wound healing was faster and of better quality in sealed areas. Partial loss of graft was at least twice as frequent in nonsealed areas.

Some authors [18] have used autologous human fibrin adhesive, thus eliminating the danger of multidonor pool preparations. The adhesive is obtained from approximately 200 ml of autologous blood. This is centrifuged and the red cells and plasma components are returned to the patients during the course of treatment or after surgery. Fibrinogen concentrate can thus be obtained and the second component of the biological adhesive, bovine thrombin, is provided. To our knowledge, there has been no case of viral transmission with fibrin glue.

A histologic study from five other patients using skin biopsies taken at days 1, 2, 5, 8, 15 and 30 was made. If fibrin glue was still present at day 2 (Fig. 3), it was completely resorbed at day 5 (Fig. 4), and there was no scar formation of signs of an inflammatory reaction. After 8 days, no difference between grafted and nongrafted areas was found.

Conclusion

In an attempt to obtain better function and appearance, minimize blood loss and increase graft survival with minimal postoperative care, we decided to treat deep burns by applying fibrin adhesive to difficult recipient sites. With fibrin glue, it is possible to reproduce, under physiological conditions, the final step of coagulation. The benefits are better: hemostasis, improved adhesion, faster healing and an antiseptic effect of the glue itself.

Unlike synthetic glues such as cryanoacrylate, biological glues are resorbable, nontoxic, do not induce an inflammatory response and promote local hemostasis in heparinized patients or patients suffering from coagulopathy.

Based on our experience, maximal benefits are obtained under the following conditions:

1. Grafts are over areas which are subject to movement (face, neck, joints, hands).
2. Grafts are not meshed for cosmetic reasons.
3. Grafts are in children.
4. Grafted area is extensive and may result in loss of skin.

References

1. Janzekovic Z (1970) A new concept in the early excision and immediate grafting in burns. J Trauma 10: 1103
2. Ihara N, Suzuki K, Tanaka H et al. (1984) Application of fibrin glue to burns: its haemostatic and skin transplants fixation effects in the excised wound. Burns Incl Therm Inj 10: 396–404
3. Rousou JA, Engleman RM, Bryer RH (1984) Fibrin glue: an effective hemostatic agent for nonsuturable intraoperative bleeding. An Thorac Surg 38: 409–410
4. Tidrick RT, Warner Ed (1944) Fibrin fixation of skin transplants. Surgery 15: 90
5. Cronkite EP, Lozner EL, Deaver J (1944) Use of thrombin and fibrinogen in skin grafting. JAMA 124: 976–978
6. Bergel S (1909) Über Wirkungen des Fibrins. Dtsch Med Wochenschr 35: 633–665
7. Brunner F (1984) Histological findings in sutured and fibrin-glued microvascular anastomosis. Arch Otorhinolaryngol 240: 311
8. Härting F, Koorneef L, Peeters HJF et al. (1985) Glued fixation of split-skin graft to the bony orbit following exenteration. Plast Reconstr Surg 76: 633–635
9. Wepner F, Fries R, Platz H (1982) The use of the fibrin adhesion system for local hemostasis in oral surgery. J Oral Maxillofac Surg 40: 555–558
10. Burnouf-Radosevich M, Duval P, Burnouf T et al. (1988) Composition protéique et qualité de colles biologiques européennes. Lyon Chir 84(2): 191
11. Redl H, Schlag G, Kuderna H et al. (1980) Biochemische Grundlagen der Fibrinklebung. Deutsch-Österreich-Schweizerische Unfalltagung in Wien 3.–6. Oktober 1979. Hefte Unfallheilkd 148: 787
12. Igisu K (1986) The role of fibronectin in the process of wound healing. Thromb Res 44: 455–465
13. Kasai S, Kunimoto R, Nitta K (1983) Cross-linking of fibrin by activated factor XIII stimulates attachment, morphological changes and proliferation of fibroblasts. Biomed Res 4: 155–160
14. Laki K, Lorand L (1948) On the solubility of fibrin clots. Science 108: 280
15. Seelich T, Redl H (1979) Das Fibrinklebersystem. Biochemische Grundlagen der Klebermethode. Dtsch Z Mund-Kiefer-Gesichts-Chir 3 [Suppl 22]
16. Woodward SC, Hermann JB, Leonard F (1964) Histotoxicity of cyanoacrylate tissue adhesives. Fed Proc (abstr) 23: 495
17. Horowitz MS, Rooks C, Horowitz B et al. (1988) Virus safety of solvent detergent treated anti-hemophilic factor concentrate. Lancet ii: 186
18. Stuart JD, Kenney JG, Lettieri J et al. (1988) Application of single-donor fibrin glue to burns. J Burn Care Rehabil 9: 619–622
19. Ronfard V, Broly H, Mitchell V et al. (1991) Use of human keratinocytes cultured on fibrin glue in the treatment of burn wounds. Burns 17: 181–184
20. Engrav LH, Heimbach DM, Walkinshaw MD et al. (1986) Excision of burns of the face. Plast Reconstr Surg 77: 744–751
21. Vibe P, Pless J (1983) A new method of skin graft adhesion. Scand J Plast Reconstr Surg 17: 263–264
22. Piechotta FU, Flemming I (1983) The maximization of wound healing with fibrin glue. Aesthetic Plast Surg 7: 81–82
23. Converse JM, Uhlschmid GK, Ballantyne DL (1969) Plasmatic circulation in skin grafts – the phase of serum inhibition. Plast Reconst Surg 43: 495
24. Vandewater L III (1985) Phagocytosis. In: McDonagh J (ed) Plasma fibronectin, structure and function. Dekker, New York, pp 175–196

Fibrin Sealant in Skin Grafting: Indications, Methods, and Pitfalls

A. Grabosch

Surgical Wound Closure

If a lesion of the skin affects all dermal layers, healing processes start, which – without surgical intervention – lead to wound closure with scar formation. To prevent infection during a lengthy period of healing or to facilitate closure in the case of more extensive defects we perform surgical wound closure. The functional and cosmetic results depend on the time of wound closure and on the chosen surgical technique.

In principal all wounds can be closed either by a suture or by split- or full-thickness skin grafts or flaps. A suture should only be done in a noninfected area and without tension using atraumatic techniques. In such cases, there is never a need for fibrin sealants; these are relevant tools in wound closure when skin grafting or flaps are required.

Indications

One can imagine the different surgical wound closure techniques as a pyramid, with the suture forming the base and the split-thickness skin graft following; we then reach the level of full-thickness skin grafts before coming to the top, represented by local or even free flaps.

If we want to close a wound area that does not show signs of infection and if we can accept a scar, then split-thickness skin grafts are indicated. This is a rather simple technique to perform, and even extensive defects, for example burns, can be covered. Furthermore, the grafts are not overly complicated.

In order to cover a limited defect on an exceptionally good wound foundation when a demanding graft is necessary, either due to functional or aesthetic reasons, a full-thickness skin graft should be used. These grafts are more demanding and, of course, only rather limited wounds can be covered.

If specific structures, such as tendons, bones, or nerves, are exposed which do not take a graft, or if the wound is insufficiently covered by a graft, perhaps because of infection, e.g., osteitis, flaps should be used. If specific tissue needs to be transferred, for example, vascularized bone or innervated muscle, a free tissue transfer using microsurgical techniques is required. Figure 1 shows the case of a young man who lost his flexor muscles in the forearm area. A free

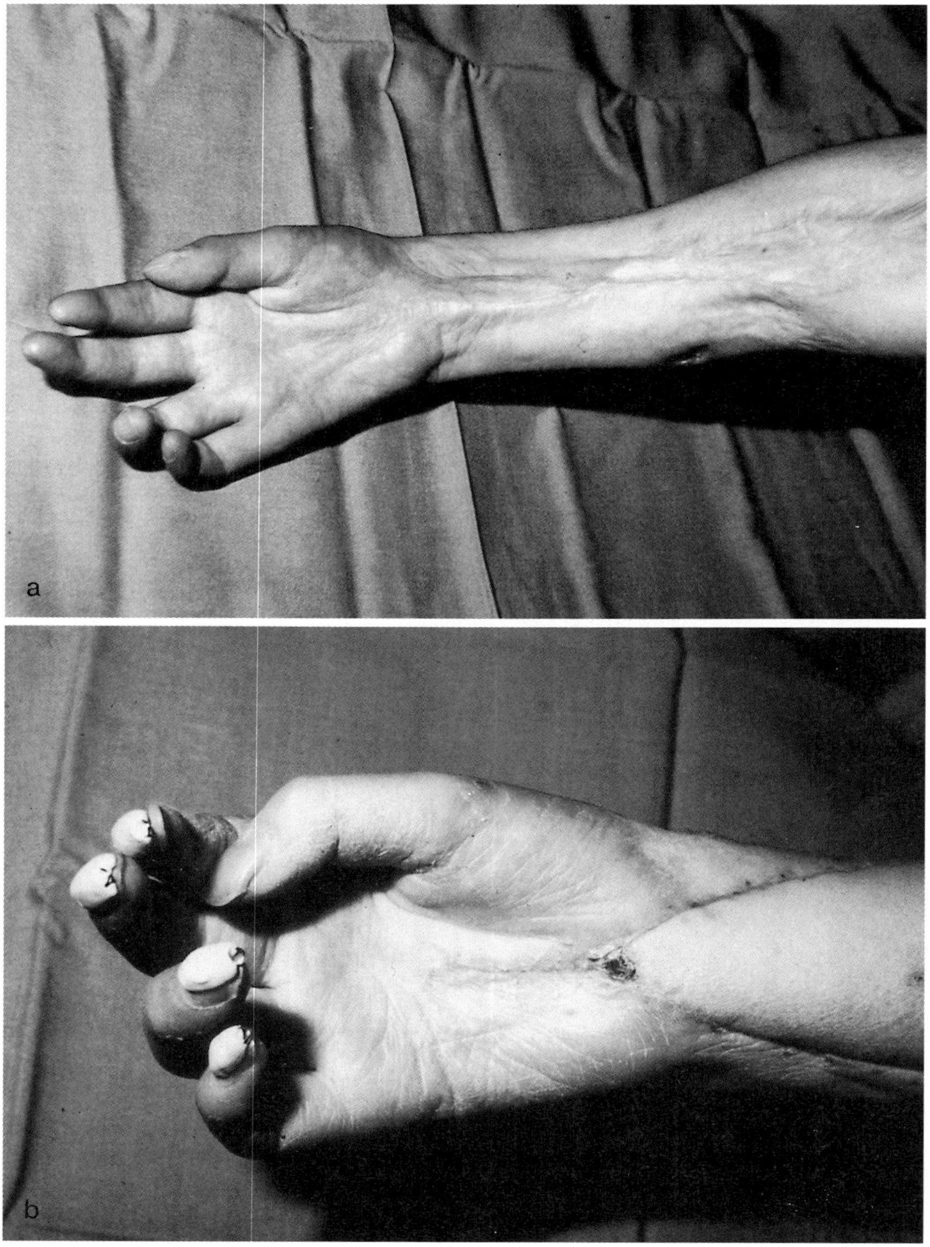

Fig. 1. a Destruction or flexor muscles; **b** function postoperatively (latissimus dorsi transfer)

latissimus dorsi muscle was transferred with a nerve suture to restore flexor function.

Surgical Techniques

Before proceeding with any type of wound closure, a very careful necrectomy must be done. If not all the infected or necrotic tissue is removed, the closure will fail. Subsequent hemostasis is also important. If a split-thickness skin graft is called for, formation of hematomas underneath the graft must be prevented. Otherwise, nourishment of the graft is disturbed due to formation of a diffusion barrier and the graft will become necrotic. Another tool to prevent hematomas and to fix the entire graft area to the wound is the application of fibrin sealant. In split-thickness skin grafts, I advise using so-called slow sealing, i. e., a sealant with a low thrombin concentration, and the spray technique (Fig. 2). This enables the surgeon to correct the position of the very thin skin graft. No further sutures are necessary to fix the graft. As a dressing we use salve-impregnated gaze, compresses, surgical cotton and gauze.

For a full-thickness skin graft, once again the wound bed must be prepared properly before placing the graft. Due to the elasticity of the full-thickness graft, it should be fixed by an additional suture. Fibrin sealant containing a high thrombin concentration is then applied with a double syringe (Fig. 4). In these cases a high thrombin concentration is desirable because the hemostatic effect is more important than fixation of the graft and extra time to place the graft is not required. With full-thickness skin grafts, a pressure dressing should always be used.

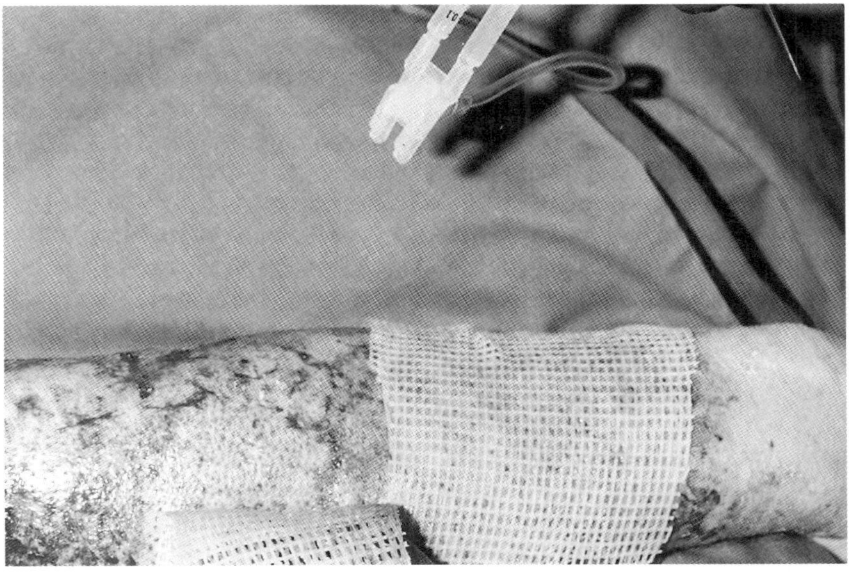

Fig. 2. Spray technique to seal split-thickness skin grafts

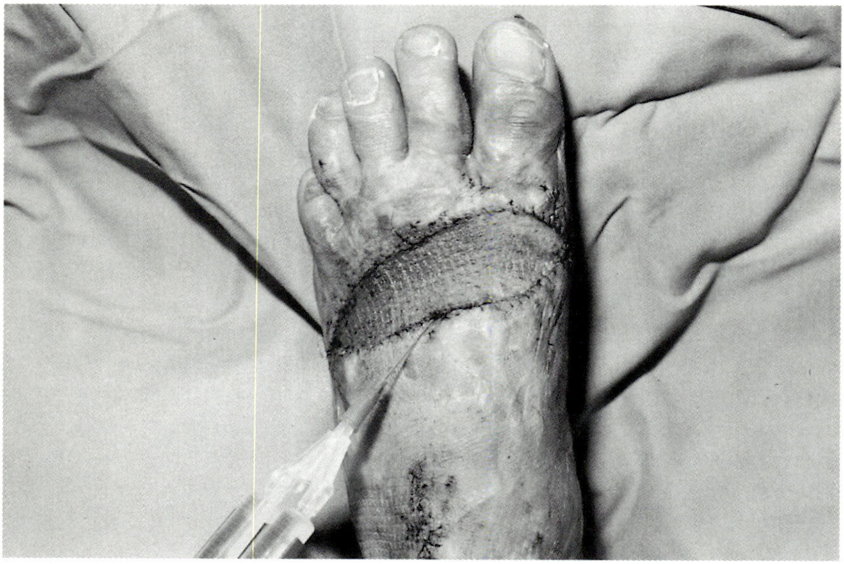

Fig. 3. Sealing full-thickness skin grafts

When doing a flap, necrectomy and hemostasis are again important. The flap, located either nearby or at another area of the body, is then placed onto the defect to be covered. It is first fixed with a few stitches to keep it in place. High thrombin concentration fibrin sealant can then be applied with double syringe. A suction drainage placed under the flap obviates the need for sealant and prevents hematomas, which can easily happen because the flap is vascularized and thus bleeding can occur from underneath or out of the flap itself.

The advantages of sealing skin grafts are a very meticulous hemostasis and less time needed for surgery, since sutures in split-thickness skin grafts are unnecessary. By fixing the whole graft to the wound base, shear forces, which will destroy the graft after the operation, are avoided. This leads to a better take rate and fewer reoperations, especially when extensive areas are grafted.

Pitfalls

If grafts or flaps are lost, either the wound base was improperly prepared or else the postoperative treatment was insufficient. Regarding the fibrin sealant, for these types of operations the fibrin layer under the graft must not be too thick. The spray technique is recommended to fix split-thickness skin grafts, and collagen sheets underneath the skin grafts should never be used.

In conclusion, the use of fibrin glue in skin grafting gives better take rates, leads to more successful clinical results, and, although it is not cheap, it is worth-while.

Cultured Autologous Keratinocytes Suspended in Fibrin Glue to Cover Burn Wounds

G. B. Stark, H. W. Kaiser, J. Kopp, and R. Horch

Abstract

The use of autologous cultured epidermal cell sheets has become a standard method for the coverage of extensively burned patients. The disadvantages of these sheet grafts are: (a) the relatively long time needed to grow the grafts, (b) technical difficulties in applying the fragile grafts resulting in an uncertain take, and (c) high costs. In a preliminary study we applied cultured keratinocytes suspended in fibrin glue onto eight burned areas in three patients with deep second and third degree burns. Glycerol-preserved, allogenic split-thickness skin was overgrafted onto this suspension four times. Reepithelialization was very rapid and ranged from 70% to 100% for overgrafted and 30% to 100% for bare keratinocyte grafts.

Histology revealed a layered squamous epithelium and indications of partial integration of allogenic dermis. Besides the good skin quality, the new technique has the advantage that it can be easily repeated and that actively proliferating epidermal cells can be transferred.

Introduction

The coverage of extensive deep burns is limited by the availability of skin graft donor sites. This is a major reason for the poor survival rates of patients with burns of more than 60%–70% total body surface area (TBSA). To circumvent the inavailability of skin graft donor sites techniques to expand autologous epidermal cells by in vitro culture have been developed [1]. Limited clinical experience with this technique has been gained using multiple layer keratinocyte sheets [2, 3]. This technique is commercially available and expensive. Further problems are an uncertain take [4] and the requirement of at least 3 weeks to produce the keratinocyte sheets. The fragile cultured grafts are difficult to handle, and nonadherence is a common problem. So far, mostly minor parts of the TBSA of major burns have been successfully covered by the sheet technique.

Keratinocyte suspensions have had limited success in wound coverage [5]. Fibrin glue appears to be a good biological support for cultured keratinocytes and protects sheet grafts [6]. Long-term results of cultured epidermal sheets after epifascial grafting have been disappointing, due to the lack of a dermal component and resulting mechanical instability.

The purpose of applying suspended epidermal cells, in contrast to cultured keratinocyte sheets, is to transplant an actively proliferating culture in vivo. This could shorten the time between harvesting and closure and improve the take rate. It is a prerequisite for treating patients with extensive burns. The new technique also aims to improve the cosmetic and functional results.

Materials and Methods

Epidermal cell culture techniques have been described by Rheinwald and Green [1] and Gallico et al. [2]: primary keratinocyte cultures are prepared from a small skin biopsy. A cell suspension is prepared from the biopsy by trypsinization and the single cells are grown on a feeder layer of lethally irradiated mouse fibroblasts. Primary cultures become confluent within 3–10 days. Then the cultures are treated again with trypsin to isolate single cells for secondary culture. On the day that the graft is to be done, the single cell suspension produced by trypsinization of 70%–80% confluent cultures is mixed with the fibrin component of fibrin glue (Tissucol, Immuno GmbH, Heidelberg, FRG). This keratinocyte-fibrinogen component is mixed with thrombin/factor XIII in the operating room and immediately applied to the wound. In two patients (four wounds) an allogenic, glycerolized split-thickness skin graft (Euro Skin Bank, Beverwijk, The Netherlands) was overlaid onto and fixed with the hardening mixture of fibrin glue and cultured keratinocytes.

Clinical Results

Wound coverage with fibrin glue keratinocyte suspensions was accomplished in eight burned areas of three patients. The patients' ages ranged form 26 to 54 years. All patients suffered deep second and third degree flame burns involving between 40% and 54% TBSA. None of the covered wounds had shown signs of spontaneous healing in response to topical treatment with silver sulfadiazine. Tangential necrectomies of the burn eschar to the deep dermis or fat were performed between day 17 and 21 after the injury. The covered wound area size ranged from 520 cm^2 to 2240 cm^2. Four wound areas were overgrafted with glycerolized allograft skin. When combined with an allograft, primary take rates within a few days ranged between 70% and 100%.

Without allograft, a continuous thin neoepidermis had completely covered the wound within 4 days. This skin was mechanically unstable and 30 cm^2 had to be regrafted after another 15 days, resulting in complete epithelialization.

When preserved cadaver skin was applied onto the keratinocyte suspension, the allograft epidermis started to dry out and desquamate about 4 days after the application. This was in contrast to the dermal component, which appeared to be integrated into a rosy new skin. The mesh graft pattern of the allograft was partially preserved. The areas covered with a combination of keratinocytes and cadaver skin remained mechanically stable and developed only minor scarring.

Additionally, two granulating burn wounds of 200 cm^2 and 600 cm^2 were grafted with the suspension without cadaver skin. The smaller of these wounds was completely epithelialized after 5 days and remained stable. The other, pretibial wound showed a primary take rate of only about 30 %, but the multiple epithelial islands formed after grafting developed a continuous skin within 2 weeks.

Histology

Nine skin biopsies from all three patients could be examined. After transplantating the keratinocyte fibrin glue suspension, a multilayer viable squamous epithelium with occasional rete ridges was seen.

When the keratinocyte suspension was overgrafted with allograft skin, epithelial cells could be seen migrating into the perforations of the mesh graft. The allogenic dermis was replaced, while the allodermis appeared to be partially integrated into the neoskin. Fibrin remnants remained discernible between the mesh and underneath the allodermis. Later after combined grafting a multilayer squamous epithelium overlaying a fibrous dermis was seen. It cannot be determined from light microscopy whether this still was composed of allograft dermis. There was a more developed rete ridge pattern than after exclusive grafting of the emulsion.

Discussion

The combination of intermingled autologous skin islands with allogenic split-thickness skin sheets (Yang et al. 1980), and the "sandwich" technique to overgraft widely meshed and expanded autologous split-thickness skin grafts with cadaver skin [7, 8], represent conventional surgical techniques to exploit the proliferative potency of epidermal cells. The cadaver skin serves as an optimal, infection-free, in vivo "culture" milieu, until the allogeneic epidermis ultimately undergoes immunogenic rejection. The fate of the cadaver dermis is much less clear [9].

Due to the restricted availability of fresh cadaver skin and possible virus transmission, glycerol preserved (nonviable) allograft skin fixed with fibrin glue has been widely used in our burn center as a routine substitute that appears to have nearly equivalent qualities [10].

Simultaneous with the development of these surgical techniques, in vitro epidermis cell culture techniques have become more sophisticated, and it has become possible to multiply keratinocytes exponentially to produce layered cultured epidermal sheets [1]. Take rates have been unpredictable, and especially third degree burns have remained problematic due to the lack of a dermal component.

It seems likely that it will soon be possible to combine the advantages of the intermingled and sandwich grafting techniques with the ready availability and proliferative potential of cultured keratinocytes.

We have added two new technical modifications to the application of autologous cultured keratinocytes: because adherence is a prerequisite for successful cell take on the wound, we added fibrin glue as a three-dimensional matrix. Transplantations of cell dispersions containing epidermocytes without a fibrin matrix have been performed previously without much success [11]. Hunyadi et al. [5] were able to heal venous ulcers with noncultured cell suspensions in fibrin glue, whereas administration without fibrin glue was without effect. Fibrin glue also improves hemostasis and has been shown to improve healing of conventional skin grafts. The application of keratinocytes in fibrin glue leads to very rapid and complete epithelialization. As is well known from cultured sheet grafts, this neoepithelium is sensitive to mechanical irritation.

As a second modification, the keratinocytes in the fibrin glue matrix were overgrafted with glycerolized cadaver grafts. Analogous to the "sandwich" technique [7], this method could be termed the "buttered swiss-cheese" sandwich technique, in which the butter corresponds to the keratinocyte-fibrin culture that fixes the meshed cadaver graft (cheese with holes). In culture, single epidermal cells exhibit a very active motility during the phases of adhesion and proliferation. So far, our clinical and histologic findings support the assumption that the suspended keratinocytes are able to migrate actively to the mesenchymal border zone to form a new layered epithelium in vivo. This shortens the in vitro culture period and avoids the very sensitive and labor intensive production steps that are necessary when sheet grafts are produced. It may also increase the cell yield, because without contact inhibition all single cells may remain able to continue vigorous proliferation in vivo.

References

1. Rheinwald JG, Green H (1975) Serial cultivation of strains of human epidermal keratinocytes; the formation of keratinizing colonies from single cells, Cell 6(3): 331–343
2. Gallico GG, O'Connor NE, Compton CC, Kehinde O, Green H (1984) Permanent coverage of large burn wounds with autologous cultured human epithelium, N Engl J Med 311(7): 448–451
3. Odessey R (1992) Multicenter experience with cultured epidermal autograft for treatment of burns, J Burn Care Rehabil 13: 174–180
4. Munster AM (ed) (1992) Cultured epidermal autograft in the management of burn patients; goals and objectives, J Burn Care Rehabil 13 (1): 123–180
5. Hunyadi J, Farkas B, Bertenyi C, Olah J, Dobozy A (1988) Keratinocyte grafting: a new means of transplantation for full-thickness wounds. J Dermatol Surg Oncol 14 (1): 75–78
6. Ronfard V, Broly H, Mitchel V, Galizia JP, Hochart D, Chambon E, Pellerin P, Huart JJ (1991) Use of keratinocytes cultured on fibrin glue in the treatment of burn wounds, Burns 17 (3): 181–184
7. Alexander JW, MacMillan BG, Law E et al. (1981) Treatment of severe burns with widely meshed skin autograft and mesh skin overlay, J Trauma 21: 433–438

8. Herndon DN, Rutan RL (1992) Comparison of cultured epidermal autograft and massive excision with serial autografting plus homograft overlay, J Burn Care Rehabil 13: 154–157
9. Kistler D, Hafemann B, Hettich R (1989) Cytogenetic investigations of the allodermis after intermingled skin grafting, Burns 15: 82
10. Horch R, Stark GB, Kopp J, Spilker G (1994) Cologne Burn Centre experiences with glycerol-preserved allogenic skin. Part I: clinical experiences and histological findings (overgraft and sandwich technique). Burns 20: 523–526
11. Billingham RE, Reynolds J (1952) Transplantation studies on sheets of pure epidermal epithelium and on epidermal cell suspensions. Br J Plast Surg 5: 52

Subject Index

Springer-Verlag and the Environment

We at Springer-Verlag firmly believe that an international science publisher has a special obligation to the environment, and our corporate policies consistently reflect this conviction.

We also expect our business partners – paper mills, printers, packaging manufacturers, etc. – to commit themselves to using environmentally friendly materials and production processes.

The paper in this book is made from low- or no-chlorine pulp and is acid free, in conformance with international standards for paper permanency.